Springer Series
in Behavior Modification
THEORY / RESEARCH / APPLICATION

Cyril M. Franks / Series Editor

Edward E. Abramson is Associate Professor of Psychology at California State University, Chico. He received his B.A. from the State University of New York at Stony Brook and his Ph.D. from the Catholic University of America. Dr. Abramson is a licensed clinical psychologist in private practice and has been on the staff of the Sutter-Yuba (California) Mental Health Services. His publications on obesity and behavior therapy have appeared in *Journal of Abnormal Psychology, Behaviour Research and Therapy, Addictive Behaviors,* and other scientific journals. Dr. Abramson has led numerous weight control groups and has conducted training programs for nurses and other health professionals.

Behavioral Approaches to WEIGHT CONTROL

EDWARD E. ABRAMSON
with contributors

SPRINGER PUBLISHING COMPANY
New York

Springer Publishing Company, Inc.
200 Park Avenue South
New York, N.Y. 10003

77 78 79 80 81 / 10 9 8 7 6 5 4 3 2 1

Library of Congress Cataloging in Publication Data

Abramson, Edward E
   Behavioral approaches to weight control.

   (Springer series in behavior modification; v. 3)
   Bibliography: p.
   1. Reducing—Psychological aspects.   2.   Behavior
modification.   3.   Food habits.   I.   Title.
[DNLM: 1.   Obesity—Therapy.   2.   Behavior therapy.
WD210 A161]
RC552.025A27   616.3'98   77–21042
ISBN 0-8261-1900-X
ISBN 0-8261-1901-8 pbk.

Printed in the United States of America

For Alina and Anne

Contents

Preface

Depending upon the estimate, there are currently between forty and eighty million Americans who are either obese or who have reason to be concerned about their weight. Until recently the only remedy for most of this population was to select one of the commonly available diets and try to muster sufficient willpower to stick to it. The results were usually disappointing. In 1967 Richard Stuart published an article outlining a behavior modification program which focused on retraining maladaptive eating habits. Instead of telling his patients which foods to eat, he taught them to alter their behavior patterns in order to make excessive eating less likely. The results of his program applied to eight female patients were impressive. Since this early report, there have been well over one hundred case reports and experimental studies of behavioral weight control programs. The vast majority of these studies report positive findings.

The widespread application of behavioral techniques has been limited because most of the relevant information has appeared in limited-circulation journals intended primarily for behavioral researchers. Furthermore, the typical research report did not describe the treatment procedures in sufficient detail to be clinically useful. Recently several excellent books on behavioral approaches to weight control have been published. A few, intended primarily for experimenters in the field, were comprised of research reports and reprinted journal articles. Others were self-help manuals directed to a general audience, or were descriptions of a single treatment program. This book has a different purpose. It was written for physicians, nurses, nutritionists, public health officials, psychologists, psychiatrists, social workers, and other professionals who will be treating overweight patients or clients. This book will provide the necessary information and materials so that the professional without extensive training in behavior modification will be able to choose and implement a behavioral treatment program.

The bulk of this book (part II) is comprised of previously unpublished treatment manuals for three behavioral programs. These manuals describe the procedures in detail since they were written for the relatively inexperienced therapist. Part III describes several additional techniques which should prove useful as adjuncts to the programs in part II.

In this book, as with any book describing therapeutic procedure in detail, there is the danger of the techniques being used in a cookbook fashion. It would be unfortunate if any set of procedures became enshrined as *the* single treatment of choice. Parts I and IV are intended to prevent this. Part I presents an overview of the etiology and traditional treatment of obesity followed by a review and appraisal of the various behavioral techniques. Part IV is a discussion of several factors which influence the effects of treatment, but are not dealt with systematically in the programs. Both parts I and IV present issues and problems which must be resolved before any program can be accepted without qualifications and modifications.

It is my hope that this book will increase the awareness of behavioral approaches to weight control on the part of concerned professionals and, in doing so, make this type of treatment available to a larger number of obese individuals.

I would like to express my appreciation to the students and colleagues who have been helpful during the preparation of this book. Specific mention should be made of Sara Armstrong-Spear's unflagging encouragement and enthusiasm. I am also grateful to Lennis Dunlap for patiently explaining to me some of the niceties of the English language and to departmental secretaries Connie Williams, Connie Cox, Deborah Murray, and Georgia Finley for tolerating a long succession of unreasonable requests. Finally, I am indebted to my wife Alina for her careful reading and thoughtful comments about the manuscript.

EDWARD E. ABRAMSON
July 1976

Contributors

EDWARD E. ABRAMSON, PH.D.
Department of Psychology
California State University, Chico
Chico, California

JEAN M. BAKER, PH.D.
Behavior Associates
Tucson, Arizona

JOSEPH R. CAUTELA, PH.D.
Department of Psychology
Boston College
Chestnut Hill, Massachusetts

EDWIN R. CHRISTENSEN, PH.D.
Murray-Jordan-Tooele Mental
  Hygiene Centro
Murray, Utah

ROY S. FOWLER, JR., PH.D.
Department of Rehabilitation
  Medicine
University of Washington
Seattle, Washington

GENEVIEVE GINSBURG, M.S.
Behavior Associates
Tucson, Arizona

D. BALFOUR JEFFREY, PH.D.
Department of Psychology
Emory University
Atlanta, Georgia

JOHN R. LUTZKER, PH.D.
Department of Psychology
University of the Pacific
Stockton, California

SANDRA Z. LUTZKER
University of the Pacific
Stockton, California

JAMES P. PAPPAS, PH.D.
Counseling and Psychological
   Services
University of Utah
Salt Lake City, Utah

JANET P. WOLLERSHEIM, PH.D.
Department of Psychology
University of Montana
Missoula, Montana

part I

introduction

1

An Overview of Etiology and Traditional Treatments

Edward E. Abramson

Adipose tissue, or fat, represents stored energy. According to one calculation, the stored energy residing in the overweight women of North America would be sufficient to provide heat and light to New York City for one year (Cappon 1973). Depending upon the measure, the prevalence of obesity in the United States is estimated at between 40 and 80 million people (Stuart and Davis 1972). In 1964 a marketing research firm found 9.5 million Americans dieting, 16.4 million watching their weight, and an additional 26.1 million who were concerned about their waistlines. The addition of an estimated 27 million who were unwilling to acknowledge their obesity resulted in a total of 79 million Americans who had reason to be concerned about their weight. This represented 58 percent of the population at that time (Wyden 1965).

Obesity can be defined as an "excessive amount of subcutaneous, nonessential fat" (Craig 1969); however, the measurement of fat and the determination of its excess are far from straightforward. Perhaps the easiest, most commonly used technique for measuring the degree of obesity is the height-weight standards which have been developed from insurance company data (e.g., Metropolitan Life Insurance Company 1959) and public health surveys (U.S. Public Health Service 1965). Using these norms, *obesity* is defined as a positive deviation of between 10 and 20 percent. Unfortunately this criterion is an indirect measure of "nonessential" fat and, therefore, has several drawbacks. For example, Behnke, Osserman, and Welham (1953) found several football players with normal fat content who would have been labeled obese on the basis of these standards. Stuart and Davis (1972) list nine other methods for determining obesity. These measures vary in complexity from the simplicity of viewing oneself nude in a mirror to various chemical and physical methods such as densitometry and isotope dilution. However, for most therapeutic purposes the height-weight norms, along with an individual's self-identification of obesity, should prove adequate.

Consequences of Obesity

The concern with the effects of obesity finds expression in the popularity of books and articles dealing with dieting and weight control, the rapid growth of weight reduction groups such as TOPS (Take Off Pounds Sensibly) and Weight Watchers, as well as in the successful marketing of numerous low-calorie and dietetic foods. Much of the interest in weight control is a consequence of the current standards of physical beauty (the wide cultural variation in attitudes toward food and standards of beauty has been described by Powdermaker [1960] among others). A second, perhaps more pressing, reason for interest in weight control is the documented evidence relating obesity to various somatic disorders. According to Kaplan and Kaplan (1957),

> the following conditions are adversely affected whenever they are associated with obesity: diabetes, heart disease, kidney disease, toxemias of pregnancy, arthritis of the spine and of the lower extremities, atherosclerosis, emphysema, cirrhosis, pulmonary embarrassment, hernia, varicose veins, post-operative thrombosis and embolus, serious accidents, obstetrical and gynecological procedures, etc. *ad infinitum.* Even fetal mortality is higher with obese women. (p. 192)

Obesity has been shown to be related, perhaps causally, to increased blood pressure, atherosclerosis, diabetes, and cancer (Kaplan and Kaplan 1957). The effects of obesity on health are illustrated by Newburgh's (1942) finding that, for men in the forty-five to fifty-five age group, there is a 1 percent increase in mortality rate for each pound of excess weight. These findings lend support to Hippocrates' earlier observation that "persons who are naturally very stout are more liable to sudden death than thin persons."

Etiology of Obesity

While a thorough discussion of the causes of obesity is beyond the scope of this chapter, several of the theories of etiology have direct implications for treatment. For the sake of convenience, the theories can be divided into two groups, biological and psychosocial. The theories need not be viewed as mutually exclusive. Obesity, like fever, may be a characteristic of more than one disorder, and may result from an interaction of biological and psychosocial factors (Welsh 1962).

Biological Theories

The theory that seems to be the most popular—that obesity is caused by metabolic factors—is the one with the least empirical support. Kaplan and Kaplan (1957) reviewed the literature and found no relationship between various metabolic factors and obesity. They also reported that glandular abnormalities could be related to fewer than 5 percent of the total number of cases of obesity surveyed.

Mayer (1968) presents a convincing argument for the role of heredity as a causal factor in obesity. He points out that heredity is readily accepted as an explanation for adiposity in animals (e.g., greyhounds tend to be leaner than bulldogs), but the same argument is rejected when applied to humans. More carefully controlled observations of the "yellow" mouse have demonstrated the existence of a genetic transmitter that causes both the yellow coat and the excessive weight characteristic of this strain.

In humans several hereditary illnesses such as Nieman-Pick and Tay Sachs diseases are characterized by abnormally large accumulations of fat in specific parts of the body. Similarly, perfectly healthy female Hottentots and Bushmen are distinguished by the unusually large fat deposits in their buttocks. Mayer suggests that it would be difficult to find plausible environmental explanations for these phenomena.

Humans cannot be used for experimental studies of genetics. Aside from the prolonged periods of time required for gestation and attaining sexual maturity, societal prohibitions against mating with a parent or sibling make this type of research impossible. As a result, most of the human research studies make use of twins. Typically, the similarities between pairs of fraternal twins are compared with the similarities between pairs of identical twins. Assuming that the twins are not separated, any greater degree of similarity of identical twins *is* presumed to be a result of the common genetic background they share. The studies cited by Mayer indicate that fraternal twins exhibit more variability in body weight than do identical twins, thus demonstrating the role of heredity in determining body weight. It appears, however, that the similarities expected on the basis of a common gene pool may not occur when the differences in environment are extreme. In other words, environmental factors may be able to overcome the genetically transmitted weight predisposition. Thus the strongest conclusion that can be drawn is that hereditary make-up may increase the likelihood of overeating or underexercising, thereby causing obesity.

A more recent theory proposes that most obesity is a function of an individual's biologically determined "set point" (Nisbett 1972). According to this view, heredity and early nutritional conditions determine the total number of fat cells. This number, fixed early in life, cannot be altered; any weight reduction must come from a decrement in the size of the cells (Hirsch and Knittle 1970). This type of obese individual who is losing weight suffers from an energy deficit and, therefore, is literally starving (Nisbett 1972). It is not surprising, then, that most obese individuals find it very difficult to adhere to low-calorie diets to maintain weight losses.

Although there is considerable variation among the biological theories, they are uniform in their implications for treatment. At the most basic level, obesity is built into the organism at birth, or shortly thereafter; as a result, attempts to lose weight are doomed to failure. This pessimistic view was stated succinctly by Mayer (quoted in Cappon 1973): "You are as curable as if you had cancer. The best way to avoid the problem is to have thin parents."

Nisbett (1972), however, cautions against premature acceptance of the inevitability of obesity. He feels that there is at least one important "weak link" in his theory and that an alternative interpretation of the research he cites is possible.

Psychosocial Theories

There is no dearth of speculation concerning various psychological and social factors presumed to cause obesity. Most of the resultant hypotheses can be lumped together under the rubric of the psychosomatic concept of obesity (Kaplan and Kaplan 1957). Much of this theorizing is based on psychoanalytic personality theory. For example, several writers (e.g., Schopbach and Matthews 1945) have characterized the mother of the obese individual as dominant and powerful, whereas the father is weak, submissive, and unable to provide guidance for the child. At least twenty-eight unconscious "meanings" of overeating have been suggested. In their review, Kaplan and Kaplan (1957) conclude:

> The present authors believe that the great number and variety indicate that *any* emotional conflict may eventually result in the symptom of overeating; it is their conclusion that the psychodynamic factors causing obesity are *non-specific*. (pp. 196–97)

They go on to explain that the common core of much of this theorizing, which is the central notion of their psychosomatic approach, is that eating serves as an anxiety-reducing mechanism for the obese. Although this view has met with widespread popular acceptance, empirical investigations yield conflicting results. In their research, Schachter, Goldman, and Gordon (1968) used the threat of painful electric shock to arouse fear. Although obese subjects were significantly more frightened than their normal-weight counterparts, their food consumption was not significantly greater. In a study designed to explore the psychosomatic concept of obesity, Abramson and Wunderlich (1972) assessed the effects of fear of electric shock and interpersonal anxiety on the eating behavior of obese and normal-weight subjects. The results were similar to those of the Schachter, Goldman, and Gordon (1968) study; the obese subjects were more responsive to the experimental manipulations (i.e., they evidenced more anxiety); however, the anxiety did not appear to affect their eating behavior. A third study (McKenna 1970), using a similar methodology, yielded conflicting results. Obese subjects consumed more food under high-anxiety conditions.

Evidence supporting the psychosomatic concept of obesity was provided by Holland, Masling, and Copley (1970). On the basis of interview data, they concluded that obese individuals eat when anxious and depressed rather than when they are hungry. Another interview study (Leon and Chamberlain 1973a) compared the eating habits of normal-weight respondents with those of obese individuals who had participated in a weight reduction group. For normals, hunger was the most frequently cited stimulus for eating. The obese, on the other hand, were more likely to choose one of several arousal states (e.g., happiness, anger, boredom, and excitement) as factors triggering eating. In an experimental study, however, Abramson and Stinson (in press) found that boredom caused increased eating for both obese and normal subjects.

Any conclusion concerning the role of emotions in the eating behavior of the obese would be premature in light of the conflicting results. Much of the difficulty stems from less than perfect research methods. Interview data are suspect because the obese may not accurately report their food consumption. The experimental studies may be inadequate since the subjects have only one type of food, typically crackers, available. Leon and Chamberlain (1973) have pointed out that this method may be inappropriate since a larger variety of more appetizing foods is available in the natural environment. Although the effects of emotions on eating are uncertain, there is considerable evidence that obese individuals are more reactive to emotional stimuli than normals (Abramson and Wunderlich 1972; Rodin 1973).

An alternative psychological approach, the external-cue hypothesis, was proposed by Schachter (1967, 1971). Essentially this view holds that eating by overweight individuals is controlled by external, cognitive, and social cues such as the taste and smell of food, the time of day, and the sight of others eating. In contrast, the food consumption of normal-weight people is a function of internal, visceral cues such as gastric motility and hypoglycemia.

The lack of correspondence between internal states and subjective feelings of hunger was first demonstrated by Stunkard and Koch (1964). Using a gastric balloon to measure stomach contractions, they found that obese subjects were almost as likely to report hunger when their stomachs were not contracting as when they were. Conversely, the obese were as likely to deny hunger when their stomachs were contracting as when they were not. In contrast, there was a relatively close correspondence between gastric contractions and reports of hunger for normal-weight subjects.

Schachter, Goldman, and Gordon (1968) had subjects report to their laboratory after missing a meal. Half of the obese group and half of the normal-weight group were fed prior to the start of the experimental task, which was rating the taste of various crackers. Deprived normals ate more than their peers who had been fed, whereas there was no difference in cracker consumption between the two obese groups. Again, eating by the obese appeared to be independent of the visceral cues that trigger eating for normal-weight individuals.

A series of ingenious studies by Schachter and his students illustrated the various external cues that can determine food consumption. For example, Schachter and Gross (1968) used doctored clocks to manipulate time. Obese subjects ate almost twice as much when they thought it was 6:05 as they did when the clock read 5:20. The role of time as an external cue regulating food consumption for the obese was supported by the results of a field study using transatlantic flight crews. The greater the weight of the flier, the less likely he was to be troubled by the discrepancy resulting from crossing time zones (i.e., the overweight flier adjusted his eating according to the local time, independent of actual food deprivation).

Ross (1969) demonstrated that cue salience affected eating by the obese. Significantly more cashew nuts were eaten when illumination was provided by a 40-watt bulb than by a 7½-watt red light.

In a study exploring the role of taste as a determinant of eating, Demke (1971) provided obese and normal-weight subjects with either a good-tasting vanilla milk shake or with a milk shake that had quinine added to it. Obese subjects drank more than normals when the milk shake was good, but drank significantly less when it had been adulterated.

Recently several investigators have demonstrated that the externality of obese individuals extends beyond the realm of food consumption. Rodin (1973) found that obese subjects, while working on tasks requiring concentration, were more distracted by competing, irrelevant material. Pliner, Meyer, and Blankstein (1974) demonstrated that obese subjects responded more strongly to positive affective stimuli than did normal-weight subjects. The clear implication of these and similar studies is that obese persons are more responsive than normals to a variety of external cues.

Both of the major psychosocial theories of the etiology of obesity have direct implications for treatment. The psychosomatic approach requires that the emotional conflict causing overeating be resolved. Bruch (1973) states: "The intrinsic task of psychotherapy aims at effecting a meaningful change in the personality so that a constructive life becomes possible without the misuse of the eating function in bizarre and irrational ways. The problem is how to achieve this" (p. 334). The effectiveness of this approach will be discussed in the next section. It should be noted, however, that a more limited interpretation of the psychosomatic concept (i.e., eating is an anxiety-reducing mechanism) has prompted at least one behavioral technique for controlling eating.

The external-cue hypothesis suggests a variety of specific techniques that have been incorporated in behavioral self-control weight reduction programs. The underlying idea is to reduce the frequency of occurrence of the various external cues that cause eating, thereby decreasing food consumption.

Traditional Treatments for Obesity

Obesity has typically been treated by medication, psychotherapy, therapeutic starvation, and reducing diets. Each treatment will be briefly reviewed.

Bruch (1973) noted that the ancient Greeks envied the Cretans who had, according to legend, a potion that enabled them to remain slender while eating as much food as they desired. Regrettably, the Cretans did not pass on their formula to present-day pharmaceutical manufacturers. Nonetheless, one of the most popular methods of weight control is the use of various prescription drugs intended to suppress the appetite. According to the Food and Drug Administration (1973), over twenty-six million prescriptions for these drugs were filled or refilled in 1971. Most of these drugs, called anorectics, contain amphetamine. The psychological effects of amphetamine include:

> wakefulness and alertness, increased initiative, elevation of mood, enhanced confidence, euphoria and elation, lessened sense of fatigue, increased motor and speech activity, and increased ability to concen-

trate. The effect on psychomotor performance is such that more work can be accomplished, but the number of errors is not necessarily decreased. (Welsh 1962, p. 59)

Many anorectics have been used as "pep pills" or misused for their stimulating effects. Unfortunately, these drugs can create dependence; heavy use may cause bizarre or psychotic behavior, and sudden withdrawal results in severe symptoms.

The utility of anorectics in weight control is debatable. Welsh (1962) offers a qualified endorsement: "There can be no question that certain anti-obesity drugs, prescribed with care, may be effective adjuncts in weight-reducing regimens" (p. 221). On the other hand, Bruch (1973) feels that amphetamines have little or no utility for promoting weight loss. She cites an early double-bind study in which the placebo treatment was as effective as the amphetamine (Bruch and Waters 1942). The Food and Drug Administration, after a review of 206 studies (FDA 1973), concluded that,

> patients receiving anorectic drugs *will* lose more weight than those who are not treated with them. But patients who take the drugs and diet will lose only a fraction of a pound more a week than those who resort only to dietary restriction. And the rate of weight loss is greatest during the early stages of taking the pills.

In summary, the most positive statement that can be made about anorectic drugs is that they *may* provide minimal short-term assistance. The short duration of any appetite-suppressing effect (typically, no longer than six weeks), combined with the very real dangers of abuse and habituation, indicates that this is not a viable treatment for obesity.

Much of the literature dealing with psychotherapy as a treatment of obesity is comprised of case reports lacking rudimentary experimental control (e.g., Lee 1955). As a result, many theoretical formulations and suggestions of techniques have been offered. Little solid evidence, however, is available to demonstrate the effectiveness of this approach to treatment. The evidence that is available is far from encouraging. For example, Holt and Winick (1961) reported the results of twenty-two sessions of psychoanalytic group therapy with six middle-class, middle-aged, obese women. The authors concluded that therapy improved the "emotional well-being" and "level of adaptation" of their patients. They also demonstrated that it was possible to predict, on the basis of edited transcripts of the therapy sessions, which patients lost weight. On the crucial issue of weight loss, however, the results were unimpressive. Thirty months after the start of the treatment, the average weight loss was 4.3 pounds. The dismal results apparently caused the analyst to alter his goals for treatment. Toward the end of the program the goal became maintenance and acceptance of weight, rather than reduction. Whatever the effects of psychotherapy may be, "uncovering conflicts alone will not prevent a person from overeating" (Berblinger 1969, p. 159).

Therapeutic starvation entails complete abstinence from food under medical supervision. Typically, patients experience the discomfort of hunger pangs for the first two to three days. Drenick (1969) stated that his patients felt that fasting was easier than dieting. After a review of the literature, Swanson and Dinello (1969) found three characteristic patterns for fasting: short-term fasts lasting no longer than two weeks, prolonged fasts lasting up to 117 days, and intermittent starvation with periods of controlled food intake. While Drenick (1969) felt that, of the three patterns, only long-term starvation holds any promise, Swanson and Dinello (1969) concluded that none of the studies they reviewed was particularly successful. They found that short-term and intermittent starvation do not promote significant weight loss or permanent change in eating habits. Long-term starvation does result in an appreciable weight loss but at the expense of psychological adjustment. The negative effects from this procedure have included paranoid reactions, infantile behavior, and increased dependency. Finally, the follow-ups of obese patients undergoing this treatment demonstrate that most will regain weight after leaving the hospital.

A comprehensive review of the innumerable programs for dietary restriction is beyond the scope of this book. Wyden (1965) presented an entertaining account of some of the more preposterous plans for painless weight loss. With dieting, as was the case with medication, the painless treatment that produces quick, permanent weight loss without altering eating habits remains to be discovered. Nonetheless, there is a considerable body of research demonstrating that calories do count; a reduction in the number of calories consumed results in decreased weight, assuming energy expenditure remains stable. The difficulty is not in finding a nutritionally sound diet that will produce weight loss, but rather in sticking to it. The average American diet has been estimated to last between sixty and ninety days, but the dieter is off the diet approximately one-half of the time. The typical weight watcher will go through this ritual approximately 1.25 times per year (Wyden 1965). Inevitably, whatever weight is lost as a result is rapidly regained. This cyclical pattern has been called the rhythm method of girth control. There is some evidence to suggest that frequent fluctuations in weight may be more harmful than constant excessive weight. According to the U.S. Public Health Service (undated), levels of serum cholesterol are elevated during weight gain. Weight loss, however, does not remove cholesterol deposits. Therefore, an individual who has had a pattern of frequent weight gains may be subject to more atherogenic stress than an individual who has been consistently obese.

In 1959 Stunkard and McLaren-Hume reviewed several hundred studies that had been reported in the medical literature over the previous thirty years. They found only eight studies that met their criteria for acceptable research design. The results of those eight studies, taken together, indicated that only 25 percent of the grossly obese were able to lose 20 pounds, while fewer than 5 percent of the patients lost 40 pounds or more. Stunkard's (1958) frequently quoted statement accurately summarizes the dismal results of the traditional treatments: "Most obese persons will not remain in treatment. Of those that remain in treatment, most will not lose weight, and of those who do lose weight, most will regain it" (p. 79).

2

Behavior Modification
in the Treatment of Obesity

Edward E. Abramson

The various behavioral treatments are based on the assumption that obesity results from excessive eating and inadequate energy expenditure. Behavior modification techniques are used to reduce or eliminate the maladaptive behaviors and to teach more appropriate behaviors. Typically, this involves overt behavior that can be observed and measured, such as drinking six ounces of cola, rather than inferred hypothetical personality states or traits (e.g., castration anxiety). However, there is some difference of opinion, even among enthusiastic proponents, regarding the specific attributes that distinguish behavior modification from other approaches to behavior change. For a brief, but comprehensive overview of the field, the reader is referred to *Behavior Modification: An Overview* by Mikulas (1972).

For our purposes, it will suffice to say that behavioral techniques are aimed at controlling the antecedents and/or consequences of various behaviors in order to change the future probability of occurrence of these behaviors (Stuart 1973). Typically, this is accomplished by the use of classical (respondent) or instrumental (operant) conditioning. In classical conditioning, a new or conditioned stimulus is paired with an unconditioned stimulus. As a result of repeated pairings, the new stimulus is able to elicit a response that previously had been elicited only by the unconditioned stimulus. Many of our emotions are thought to have been acquired in this fashion (Wolpe 1973). In operant conditioning, the contingent presentation of certain events (e.g., reinforcers such as money) following the occurrence of a specific behavior has the effect of changing the probability that the behavior will be repeated in the future.

In an earlier review (Abramson 1973) I divided the various behavioral techniques into five categories: aversive conditioning, covert sensitization, coverant conditioning, therapist reinforcement of weight loss, and self-control of eating. The addition of several new approaches, and variations upon earlier techniques, has had the effect of creating a confusing array of different strategies, all falling within the general heading of behavior modification. Figure 2-1 is a hierarchical ordering that should be useful in clarifying the conceptual relationships between these techniques.

Respondent Methods

This approach to weight control relies exclusively on aversive conditioning to decrease the amount of food consumed. Typically, an aversive stimulus is presented simultaneously with a food stimulus. After repeated pairings, the food stimulus should arouse the same unpleasant sensations elicited by the aversive stimulus, thus decreasing the attractiveness and consumption of the food. This procedure is called aversion therapy when the pairings are presented in reality, and covert sensitization when they are presented in imagination.

Aversion Therapy

An early example of this technique was provided by Moss (1924). A clicking noise was paired with vinegar consumption. After repeated pairings, the child who was the subject of this study rejected orange juice when it was presented with the same noise. A more commonly used aversive stimulus is electric shock. Shock has been paired with verbally presented images of desirable foods (Wolpe 1954), with the subject's physical movement toward a desir-

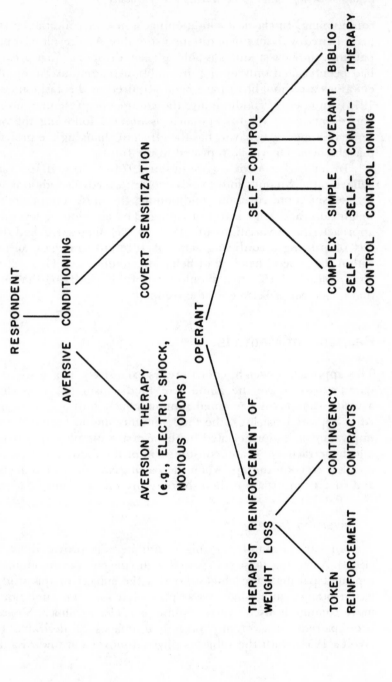

Figure 2-1 Behavioral Techniques for Treating Obesity

able food presented by the experimenter (Meyer and Crisp 1964), and with the subject's verbalization of a stimulus word, *overeating* (Thorpe et al. 1964). Of the four subjects in these reports, three did not remain in treatment (Wolpe's subject died from unrelated causes), while the fourth lost a significant amount of weight. An experimental study comparing an aversive procedure similar to that used by Wolpe with several other procedures also yielded discouraging results. After eight weeks of treatment, aversive therapy did not result in significant weight loss (Stollak 1967).

The noxious odor of butyric acid has been used as an aversive stimulus by Kennedy and Foreyt (1968). In their case study, the subject lost 30 pounds. The authors note, however, that their treatment had the effect of increasing the consumption of nontarget foods (i.e., foods that were not paired with the noxious odor). They attributed the successful weight loss to other techniques that were being used concurrently. This procedure was compared with a control procedure in a later experimental study (Foreyt and Kennedy 1971). Although the subjects undergoing the aversion therapy treatment lost more weight than control subjects (13 pounds versus 1 pound), the authors felt that the relationship that developed between the subject and the therapist played a major role in producing the weight loss. Therefore, the results of the study did not allow any firm conclusions to be drawn regarding the effectiveness of aversion therapy by itself. A recent study using a variation of this approach was more successful. Morganstern (1974) used cigarette smoke as the aversive stimulus paired with the act of eating various problem foods. The subject was a nonsmoker who reported that smoking produced unpleasant sensations including nausea and dizziness. Data were presented demonstrating sharp declines in the consumption of the various target foods, as well as a 41-pound weight loss by the end of the eighteen weeks of treatment. Although this case study had a single subject, the use of a multiple-baseline design (Baer, Wolf, and Risley 1968) allows limited conclusions to be drawn from the findings. For this subject, the aversive conditioning, rather than uncontrolled, nonspecific factors, was responsible for the altered eating behavior and weight loss. It should be noted that Morganstern does not feel that the technique is likely to promote adaptation to cigarette smoking.

Tyler and Straughan (1970) used breath-holding as an aversive stimulus which was paired with imagined presentations of desirable foods. After seven weeks of treatment, the average weight loss for the participants was 0.43 pounds.

Despite the occasional positive outcome with aversion therapy, a well-controlled experimental study demonstrating significant weight loss is lacking. The earlier conclusion that "despite some early enthusiasm, there is little evidence to indicate that aversive procedures are an effective treatment for obesity" (Abramson 1973) still seems appropriate.

Covert Sensitization

This technique was first proposed by Cautela (1966, 1967). The patient is relaxed first. The therapist then verbally presents vivid scenes, described at some length, in which the patient approaches a problem food, starts to eat the food, becomes violently ill, and vomits. This sequence is repeated several times with successful avoidance scenes. In the avoidance scenes, the patient approaches the target food, begins to feel nauseated, retreats from the food, and feels an immediate sense of relief. Recently, Maletzky (1973) introduced a procedure he calls "assisted" covert sensitization, which adds components of aversion therapy to covert sensitization. While presenting the aversive scenes verbally, the therapist introduces a highly unpleasant odor (valeric acid). He reported success in treating one obese patient.

Although Cautela claims that "Of all the syndromes treated, covert sensitization seems to be most effective in dealing with the problems of obesity" (1967, p. 463), the experimental studies using this technique report conflicting findings. Janda and Rimm (1972) found that six sessions of covert sensitization resulted in an average weight loss of 9.5 pounds, which was increased to 11.7 pounds at the six-week follow-up. The control and attention-placebo groups demonstrated either a trivial weight loss or weight gain at the follow-up. An additional positive finding was the high correlation ($r = .53$) between weight loss and ratings of subjective discomfort caused by the treatment. This suggests that aversive conditioning rather than some nonspecific factor was responsible for the successful weight loss. In a study comparing six sessions of covert sensitization with an equal number of covert positive reinforcement sessions and a control treatment, Manno and Marston (1972) found the two covert conditioning treatments were equally effective. Three months after treatment, the

mean weight loss was 8.9, 8.9, and 5.2 pounds for the covert reinforcement, covert sensitization, and control groups respectively. In a
less well-controlled study, Murray and Harrington (1972) reported
an average weight loss of 5.9 pounds for female subjects completing
ten weeks of a covert sensitization treatment.

Meynen (1970) compared eight sessions of covert sensitization
with an equal number of sessions devoted to a modified systematic
desensitization procedure, a relaxation treatment, and a no-treatment control. The three treatments were significantly more effective
than the control although they did not differ significantly from each
other. Since all of the active treatments included dietary information, weekly weigh-ins, and monitoring of eating behavior, it is
difficult to assess the specific contributions of the covert sensitization
to the weight losses.

Negative outcomes were reported in several studies. Harris
(1969) added three weeks of covert sensitization to a behavioral self-
control program that had lasted two months. No additional weight
loss occurred. Lick and Bootzin (1971) found that two covert sensitization treatments (differing only in the explanation for treatment
that was given to the subjects) were not significantly more effective
than the no-treatment control. One consequence of treatment was
that subjects changed their ratings of the attractiveness of various
fattening foods. Although the rated attractiveness of these foods
declined, many subjects continued to eat them. The others, who
decreased their consumption of these foods, did not lose weight
because they increased their intake of other foods. A final finding,
that there was no relationship between discomfort during treatment
and weight loss, contradicts Janda and Rimm's (1972) results.

Several studies have assessed the relative importance of the various components of the covert sensitization technique. Manno (1972)
compared five covert treatments, including two that lacked aversive
scenes. The nonaversive treatments were more effective than those
with the aversive imagery. Sachs and Ingram (1972) compared the
effectiveness of covert sensitization with a covert procedure that involved backward conditioning (i.e., the aversive vomit scene was presented first, followed by the pleasurable food imagery). The two
procedures were equally effective in reducing consumption of target
foods. This finding is inconsistent with the learning theory rationale
for covert sensitization. Therefore, it was suggested that motiva-
tional factors, rather than aversive conditioning, are responsible for

the results obtained with covert sensitization. In a similar study, Foreyt and Hagen (1973) compared eighteen sessions of covert sensitization with a no-treatment control and a covert placebo treatment. The latter treatment involved the presentation of pleasant scenes (e.g., lying in an open field among colorful flowers) interspersed between eating scenes. On the basis of the learning rationale for covert sensitization, it would be predicted that the covert placebo treatment would result in *increased* attractiveness and consumption of target foods. The results indicated no differences in weight change between groups. However, the subjects undergoing both of the covert treatments reported significant decreases in their liking of favorite foods after treatment. The authors also mention anecdotal reports provided by the subjects indicating that the covert placebo treatment was effective in modifying food preferences (e.g., one subject became sick after forcing herself to eat a hamburger). Since conditioning cannot account for these results, it was concluded that suggestion was responsible for the effects of the covert placebo treatment. It was inferred, therefore, that the results of covert sensitization may be attributed to nonspecific factors such as attention and suggestion rather than aversive conditioning as originally proposd.

Recently, Elliott and Denney (1975) and Diament and Wilson (1975) have provided evidence indicating that any beneficial effects of covert sensitization result from placebo or other nonspecific factors. Elliott and Denney (1975) compared three treatments: attention-placebo and covert sensitization treatments that were similar to those used by Manno and Marston (1972) and a covert sensitization plus false feedback treatment. Subjects in the latter treatment were told that the bogus biofeedback data they received were a measure of the effects of treatment. All three treatments produced equivalent weight loss. The only differences reported were in desirability of target foods. The false feedback led to greater reduction in desirability in comparison with the covert sensitization treatment without feedback.

In what is perhaps the most damaging study, Diament and Wilson (1975) replicated Foreyt and Hagen's (1973) experiment by comparing a covert sensitization treatment with a covert placebo and no treatment. In addition to the usual measure of weight lost, target food consumption in an analogue eating situation and an objective measure of food palatability were the dependent variables. The analogue was a taste-rating task similar to that used by Schachter, Goldman, and Gordon (1968) and others. Palatability was assessed by measuring salivation during periods of imagery involving the consumption of the target food (Wooley and Wooley 1973). The inclusion of these dependent variables provides a more precise measure of the specific effects of covert sensitization (Abramson 1973). None of the objective measures showed differences between the three treatment groups.

As Diament and Wilson (1975) point out, it is impossible to prove the null hypothesis (i.e., covert sensitization does *not* work). The accumulating evidence, however, has been negative.

Operant Methods

The strategy of operant methods is to systematically attach consequences to target behaviors in order to modify the probability of the behavior occurring again. Although the basic principles being applied are the same, an important practical distinction can be made on the basis of who controls the consequences, the therapist or his client (i.e., self-control).

Therapist Reinforcement of Weight Loss

There have been several reports in which reinforcement contingencies, applied in an institutional setting, resulted in significant weight loss. In the first such study (Ayllon 1963), the patient was removed from the hospital dining hall when she approached tables other than her own, or ate food belonging to others. After two weeks the problem behavior, food stealing, stopped and the patient's weight gradually declined. Moore and Crum (1969) used attention and praise to reinforce weight losses achieved by a chronic schizophrenic resident of a large mental institution. The patient lost 35 pounds over a twenty-eight-week interval. In an experimental study, Harmatz and Lapuc (1968) compared the effectiveness of a behavior modification treatment with group therapy and diet-only treatments. In the behavior modification group, hospitalized subjects lost a portion of their $5 weekly allowance if they did not exhibit a weight loss at the weekly weigh-in. After six weeks of treatment, both the behavior modification and group therapy treatments had produced greater weight losses than the diet-only treatment. A follow-up four weeks later revealed that the behavior modification patients exhibited significantly greater weight losses than patients in the other two groups.

Three case reports (Bernard 1968; Upper and Newton 1971; Klein et al. 1972) demonstrated the utility of reinforcement procedures conducted within the context of a token-economy psychiatric ward. Typically, patients were given tokens and social reinforcement or extra privileges for attaining specified weight reduction goals. The eight patients described in the three studies achieved clinically significant weight losses.

In all of the studies described above, it was relatively easy for the therapist to control the dispensing of reinforcers since, to a large extent, the therapist controlled the patient's total environment (i.e., the hospital ward). Application of therapist-controlled reinforcement in a natural environment is more difficult because of the therapist's limited influence. Dinoff, Rickard, and Colwick (1972) described a contingency-contracting procedure which was used with an emotionally disturbed ten-year-old boy attending a summer camp. Basically, a contingency contract is an agreement between two or more individuals specifying that certain reinforcers will be forthcoming only when the agreed-upon objective (in this case, weight loss) is attained. The subject of this study lost 30 pounds during the seven-week camping session.

A similar technique for controlling reinforcers in the natural environment was described by Tighe and Elliot (1968). This approach requires that the client deposit money or other valuable items with the therapist at the start of treatment. The client is reinforced by getting back a portion of his money or valuables each time he reaches a previously agreed-upon goal. The applicability of this technique to weight control was demonstrated by Mann (1972). A contract was signed which specified the subject's final weight reduction goal, as well as the number of pounds to be lost during each two-week period of treatment. Eight subjects were used in this experiment, each serving as her own control. When the contingencies were in operation (i.e., the subject lost her valuables for failing to meet the goal), the average weight loss was 2.1 pounds per week during the first treatment period and 1.2 pounds per week during the second. On the other hand, when the contingencies were not in effect, subjects gained an average of from 0.9 to 1.9 pounds per week. This suggests that the contingency, rather than any extraneous variable, was responsible for the weight loss. Although five of the subjects were able to reach their goal, and the remaining three made significant progress toward their goals, this technique was not without problems. Since the target was weight, rather than eating behavior, several subjects used laxatives and diuretics to promote rapid weight loss. While the terms of the contract were satisfied, it is unlikely that use of these medications would result in long-term weight loss. In a later study, Mann (1973) acknowledged that some of the subjects began to regain weight after the termination of treatment. Jeffrey, Christensen, and Pappas (1972) reported similar results. Four subjects participating in a treatment program in which a contingency contract played a major role exhibited a mean weight loss of 27 pounds. However, six months after treatment, one subject had returned to his original weight, while the second had regained a major portion of the weight he had lost. A possible solution to this problem was suggested by Mann (1973). Basically, he proposed an indefinite extension of the contract. Although this would have the effect of keeping the patient in therapy, he pointed out that this procedure would require only five minutes of a therapist's or paraprofessional's time per week.

Lutzker and Lutzker (1974), a husband and wife team, used less artificial contingencies to promote the wife's weight loss. Weekly weight loss of ½ pound or more resulted in her receiving a predetermined reinforcer of her choice. Stable weight caused a forfeiture of the reinforcer, while weight gain resulted in a lack of reinforcement and punishment, i.e., the husband was not responsible for his share of the household chores during the following week. The subject lost 7½ pounds during the first eight-week treatment period, gained 1½ pounds when the contract was temporarily suspended, and then lost an additional 3½ pounds when the contract was reinstated. She maintained a 14-pound weight loss for the year following treatment.

In an experimental study, Christensen and Barrios (1975) collected a monetary deposit from overweight participants. Each week, they were randomly paired and encouraged to meet with each other in order to provide advice and encouragement. At the weekly weigh-in, partial return of the deposit was contingent upon the weight loss of both partners. At the end of the five-week treatment, the results were significantly better than those of control groups although not clinically significant. The authors feel that the group contingency was more effective than a comparable individual contingency would have been. Unfortunately, no permanent social support developed. During the follow-up period in which there were no contingencies, there was considerable deterioration of treatment effects, suggesting that some type of long-term contingency is required to maintain weight losses.

Aragona, Cassady, and Drabman (1975) used contingency contracts with the parents of overweight girls (aged five to ten). The parents were taught self-control techniques to apply to their daughters. The contingency contract for the response-cost group required that parents deposit specified sums of money with the experimenters at the start of treatment. Failure to attend meetings, complete assignments, or lose weight resulted in forfeiture of part of the deposit. Parents in the response-cost plus reinforcement group agreed in addition to provide weekly reinforcement to the child for weight loss. After twelve weeks of treatment, both treatments resulted in significantly more weight loss than a no-treatment control. At the eight-week follow-up, the response-cost plus reinforcement treatment was superior to the response-cost-only treatment, but this difference disappeared at the thirty-one-week follow-up.

While it is relatively easy for a therapist to reinforce weight loss in an institutional setting, outpatient treatment is more difficult. With the patient's cooperation, contingency contracts can be used to provide therapist-controlled reinforcement. However, the long-term effectiveness of therapist-controlled reinforcement inside and outside institutions remains to be demonstrated. This procedure does not teach the patient new methods of decreasing food consumption or increasing exercise. Instead, the patient must rely on previously learned techniques such as dieting or skipping meals in order to fulfill the terms of the contract. In most instances these techniques are likely to be aversive to the patient, who, as a result, may stop using them upon the termination of treatment.

Complex Self-Control

There is some confusion, even in the behavioral literature, regarding the meaning of the term *self-control*. Most frequently it is confused with *willpower*. Willpower, according to Mahoney and Thoresen (1974) is a "vaguely defined inner force." The term is used only after the fact. Thus, if an individual is unsuccessful in controlling his eating, we accuse him of lacking willpower. However, this process does not clarify the problem. It does not suggest any specific strategy for rectifying the situation. The only consequence of this process is to convince everyone involved of the inevitability of continued excessive eating. In contrast, self-control refers to any of a large variety of specific techniques that an individual can use to modify his own behavior. Thus the term *self-control,* as used here, does not refer to a vague inner force or personality trait, but rather to "the identification and control of specific environmental events that affect specific behaviors" (Williams and Long 1975, p. 4).

The behavioral rationale and suggested techniques for self-control treatments of obesity were first presented by Ferster, Nurnberger, and Levitt (1962). They theorized that the act of putting food into one's mouth is immediately reinforced by a variety of pleasant sensations, while the aversive consequences of overeating (i.e., weight gain) occur at some unspecified time in the future. Therefore, the immediate reinforcers are more potent determinants of behavior. To alter this pattern, the authors suggest four steps: determining the variables affecting eating, manipulating these variables, identifying the aversive consequences of eating, and developing a plan for the successive approximations of the desired behaviors.

Treatment was conducted in group sessions. Much of the time was devoted to developing a repertoire of individual aversive consequences for overeating. Each participant was encouraged to be explicit in describing specific situations in which being overweight was aversive. Subjects kept a written record of their food consumption. Environmental manipulations intended to reduce the number of stimuli triggering eating were suggested. Although the results of treatment were not reported, Stunkard (1972) characterized the outcome as "poor." A similar rationale for a self-control treatment was presented by Goldiamond (1965) with a brief example.

Stuart's (1967) article was the first to provide outcome data for a behavioral self-control program. In contrast with the procedures outlined by Ferster, Nurnberger, and Levitt (1962), the aversive consequences of overeating were deemphasized. Eight female patients attended between nineteen and forty-one individual sessions. Weight loss over the course of a year ranged from 26 to 47 pounds, which was characterized by Stunkard (1972) as "the best results ever obtained in office treatment of obesity" (p. v). This report, which included an outline for twelve therapeutic interviews, provoked considerable interest and additional research. In more recent work (Stuart 1971; Stuart and David 1972), techniques were included for increasing energy expenditure and nutritional management.

The first of several controlled experimental studies was conducted by Harris (1969). A no-treatment control group was compared with two self-control groups. The experimental groups met twice weekly for two months. Three types of techniques for controlling food consumption were taught to the participants: self reward for refraining from eating, decreasing the number of stimuli that tend to elicit eating, and altering the actual behaviors that are involved in food consumption (e.g., chewing food slowly and leaving small amounts of food on the plate). All experimental subjects lost weight, and the difference between control and experimental groups was significant (control subjects gained an average of 3.6 pounds, while experimental subjects lost an average of 10.5 pounds).

In an elegantly controlled study, Wollersheim (1970) compared a behavioral group treatment with a no-treatment control, a nonspecific treatment, and a positive-expectation–social-pressure treatment. All treatments involved ten sessions over the course of three months. Each group was comprised of five participants (female college students 10 percent or more overweight). Each of the four therapists (two men and two women) led one of each type of group, thus controlling the possible confounding influence of the therapist's sex or personality upon treatment outcome. To ensure uniformity, a highly specific treatment manual was prepared for each type of treatment.

The positive-expectation–social-pressure group was an attempt to replicate the procedures of TOPS and other self-help groups. A clear expectation of weight loss was communicated to the participants, and social pressure was manipulated to provide motivation for weight reduction. The nonspecific treatment was devoted to discussion of underlying "personality make-up" and "unconscious motives" that were responsible for obesity. Muscle relaxation was also used, ostensibly to help develop insights. The behavioral treatment involved some manipulation of social pressure and positive expectation. Muscle relaxation was taught with the rationale that it would be useful to counter tension in situations where tension typically provoked eating. The unique aspect of this treatment, however, was the functional analysis of each participant's eating behavior. Each eating record was reviewed in order to develop stimulus control of eating. Additional techniques included self-reinforcement for controlling eating, establishing alternative reinforcers to be used instead of food, and aversive imagery.

The three treatments yielded a significantly greater weight reduction than the control. The behavioral treatment, however, was significantly more effective than the nonspecific or the positive-expectation–social-pressure treatments, which did not differ. A follow-up eight weeks later showed slight increases in weight for all participants, but the behavioral group still showed a significantly greater weight loss than the other groups. Using a criterion of 9 pounds for a "significant" weight loss, the data indicate that 6 percent of the controls, 25 percent of the positive-expectation–social-pressure, 40 percent of the nonspecific, and 61 percent of the behavioral group exhibited significant reductions. At the follow-up, the behavioral group remained the most effective.

Penick et al. (1971) compared the effectiveness of a behavior modification group with a traditional therapy group. The thirty-two subjects were participants in a day-care program for the treatment of obesity. Both groups, in sessions lasting about two hours, were co-led by a male and female therapist. The traditional treatment involved supportive psychotherapy, nutrition and dieting information, and, upon demand, appetite-suppressing medication. The behavioral treatment was similar to that used by Ferster, Nurnberger, and Levitt (1962) and Stuart (1967). After three months of treatment, 33 percent of the behavioral group lost more than 30 pounds while 53 percent exhibited weight losses greater than 20 pounds. By the one-year follow-up, 40 percent of the participants had reached the higher criterion. A comparison with the traditional treatment group yielded statistically significant differences using the 30-pound criterion.

Stuart (1971) tested his three-dimensional program (diet and exercise management were added to the behavioral self-control procedures) using a crossover design. After a five-week period in which participants kept eating and weight records but did not receive any treatment, two groups of three participants were formed. The first group participated in the three-dimensional program for fifteen weeks, while the second was given the diet-planning and exercise-management materials only. At the end of the fifteen weeks, members of the first group were asked to continue using the procedures they had learned while the three-dimensional program was instituted for the second group. Three months after the second group had completed treatment, weight loss averaged 35 pounds for the first group and 21 pounds for the second. The fact that the second group did not start to lose weight until the beginning of the three-dimensional treatment suggests that the treatment, rather than nonspecific factors, was responsible for weight loss. Stuart's program was also tested by Balch and Ross (1974). Nineteen subjects participated in a nine-week group treatment which revolved around a didactic presentation of the material covered in the condensed version of Stuart's (1972b) book. The results were compared with those obtained from a no-treatment control and a group of subjects who started, but failed to complete, the group treatment. The full-treatment group lost significantly more (an average of 10.6 pounds) than either of the other groups. A six-week follow-up indicated that thirteen of the nineteen participants completing treatment were able to maintain their weight loss or make further progress.

In most of these studies, subjects were recruited for the sole purpose of participating in an experiment. It could be argued that the idea of participating in research creates the expectation of a new powerful treatment. The results of the studies could be partially attributed to the subjects' expectancies rather than to the actual effects of the treatment procedures. Several recent studies have reported the effects of self-control techniques when added to an ongoing treatment program. These studies have the advantage of testing self-control programs in a more realistic setting as well as including a larger number of subjects.

Levitz and Stunkard (1974) made use of sixteen chapters of TOPS to compare a self-control program conducted by mental health professionals with a similar program led by trained TOPS leaders and a continuation of the usual TOPS program. The behavioral groups had a lower attrition rate and lost more weight during the three-month treatment period than the standard TOPS group. At the nine-month follow-up, these differences had increased. The professionally led groups lost significantly more weight than the behavioral groups led by TOPS leaders. The authors note, however, that weight losses were not as great as those reported in some of the earlier research.

Musante (1976) reported the results of the Dietary Rehabilitation Clinic at Duke University. This is an intensive behavioral program that includes medical and dietary components. All of the 229 obese patients had a history of unsuccessful prior attempts at weight reduction. The average length of treatment was 10.4 weeks for women and 8.2 weeks for men. Weight loss averaged 2.3 and 3.5

pounds per week for women and men, respectively. Over one-half of the patients lost 20 or more pounds while about one-quarter lost 40 or more pounds. These results compare favorably with the previously cited research although no follow-up data are reported.

The results of the treatment of sixty-two patients at the Stanford University Eating Disorders Clinic were reported by Ferguson (1976). The program, which includes maintenance periods, lasts a total of forty weeks. After ten weeks of treatment, 93 percent had lost some weight while 40 percent lost 10 pounds or more. The average weight loss was 9.7 pounds. There were considerable differences between patients in weight loss and between therapists in treatment effectiveness.

In summary, the efficacy of behavioral self-control programs for weight reduction has been demonstrated in clinical settings with patients representative of the obese population. Self-control programs are not without problems, however. Some of these concerns will be discussed in part IV.

Components of Self-Control Programs

In light of the favorable results reported in the various outcome studies, researchers have recently devoted their attention to conducting studies designed to determine which are the critical components of self-control programs, and which, if any, are superfluous. One component of most self-control programs, self-monitoring, has been the subject of several experimental studies. Romanczyk (1974) contrasted weight losses of a no-treatment control with treatments comprised of self-recording of daily weight, self-recording of daily weight and daily caloric intake, behavior management instructions without self-recording, and behavior management with self-recording of both daily weight and daily caloric intake. At the end of the initial four-week treatment period, there was no difference between the no-treatment control and the self-monitoring of daily weight groups. The major finding of the study, however, was that self-recording of daily weight and daily caloric intake (without therapist contact) was as effective as the behavior management and behavior management with self-recording treatments. Both of these groups had weekly therapist contact. Romanczyk suggests that the failure to find weight loss attributable to the self-control procedures, above that caused by self-monitoring, may be due to a "floor effect." Given the relatively brief duration of treatment, participants could not have exhibited a more rapid weight loss without a drastic decrease in food consumption. Nonetheless, the findings strongly suggest that self-monitoring of daily caloric intake is a significant component of behavioral self-control treatments.

The most comprehensive study of the components of behavioral treatment was performed by Romanczyk et al. (1973). Seven groups were used to assess the relative effectiveness of the following behavioral techniques: self-monitoring, covert sensitization, relaxation training, self-control, and therapist reinforcement. The major finding of this study was that self-monitoring of daily caloric intake was as effective as any of the more complex techniques, either individually or in combination. As a result of the experimental design used in this study, it was not possible to make a follow-up comparison of self-monitoring with the more complex behavioral techniques. Again, the "floor effect" and the short duration of treatment (four weeks) may have served to attenuate differences between treatments. A second experiment was conducted to allow for a follow-up comparison between self-monitoring and a combination behavioral treatment including all of the component techniques listed above. While both groups produced significant weight loss at the end of treatment, the complex behavioral treatment was significantly more effective. This difference was maintained at the three- and twelve-week follow-ups, providing additional support for the superiority of the full treatment package.

Bellack, Rozensky, and Schwartz (1974) compared the effects of several forms of self-monitoring on eating behavior. Three treatment groups, using Stuart's (1971) format, were compared with a no-treatment control group. The groups differed only in that the first was instructed to record food intake before consumption (premonitoring), the second recorded after consumption (postmonitoring), while the third group did not make use of self-monitoring. The premonitoring treatment was most effective; every participant lost weight. Interestingly, both the premonitoring and nonmonitoring groups continued to lose weight after the completion of treatment, while the postmonitoring group did not differ from the untreated control group. The results suggest that monitoring can be an effective component of treatment if the recording occurs prior to food intake, but may decrease the effectiveness of treatment if recording is done after eating.

In two studies, Mahoney and his associates explored the role of self-reward and self-punishment in producing weight loss. Mahoney, Moura, and Wade (1973), using five groups, compared the effects of self-reward, self-punishment, a combination of both, self-monitoring, and a control. All groups (including the control) received booklets describing stimulus-control approaches to weight reduction. Self-reward and self-punishment participants were instructed to award or fine themselves a part of their monetary deposits contingent upon weight loss or other desirable or undesirable eating-related behaviors. The self-imposed rewards and/or punishments were meted out at the biweekly weigh-ins. Self-monitoring subjects participated in the weigh-ins but did not reward or punish themselves. Following four weeks of treatment, self-reward subjects had lost significantly more weight than either the self-monitoring or control subjects, while self-punishment subjects did not differ significantly from any of the other groups. Four months later an analysis of the data indicated that the self-reward group and the self-reward plus self-punishment group had lost significantly greater percentages of their body weight than the information-control group. These findings were interpreted as suggesting that self-reward for desirable behaviors is more effective than either self-punishment for undesirable behaviors or self-monitoring. It should be noted, however, that the type of self-monitoring procedure was not specified. Thus, it is possible that participants recorded their food intake after consumption, which has been shown to be ineffective (Bellack, Rozensky, and Schwartz 1974).

In a follow-up study, Mahoney (1974) compared a self-monitoring treatment with a self-reward for weight loss treatment, a self-reward for eating habit improvement treatment, and a control. The results, both at termination of treatment and two months later, indicate that self-reward was superior to self-monitoring, and that self-rewards for changes in eating habits are more effective than self-rewards for weight loss.

The superiority of self-reinforcement to self-monitoring was further demonstrated by Bellack (1976). In contrast to Mahoney's studies, self-monitoring subjects were specifically instructed to do their recording *before* eating. Despite this strengthening of the self-monitoring, self-reinforcement resulted in significantly greater weight loss.

Finally, McReynolds et al. (1976) compared a typical behavioral self-control package which included the usual array of techniques with a simpler program based almost exclusively on the stimulus control techniques. The latter treatment, based on Schachter's external-cue hypothesis, included a variety of suggestions intended to reduce the cues that trigger eating. Both groups exhibited equal weight losses at the end of treatment. The stimulus control treatment was superior at both the three- and six-month follow-ups. The clear implication is that many of the components of the typical self-control program are unnecessary and perhaps counterproductive. This finding is difficult to reconcile with recent challenges to external-cue hypothesis (e.g., Mahoney 1975*a*). If this finding is replicated, self-control programs should be revised to place a greater emphasis on the stimulus control techniques.

Bibliotherapy

The influence of the therapist in behavioral self-control groups has been investigated in several studies. Typically, these studies have contrasted a leader-led behavioral group with a bibliotherapy group. The latter treatment makes use of a manual outlining the various behavioral principles and procedures. The success of the leaderless bibliotherapy treatments warrants their discussion as a separate treatment approach.

Hagen (1974) made use of Wollersheim's behavioral program. The bibliotherapy group received a revised version of Wollersheim's treatment manual in ten weekly installments. There was no therapist contact; manuals were distributed, and homework was returned through the mail. A second group made use of the manual, but the exchange of lessons took place at weekly therapy sessions lasting one hour. The third and fourth groups were a replication of Wollersheim's therapist-led behavioral group and a no-treatment control group. The three experimental treatments produced significantly greater weight losses than the control, but there were no significant differences between the three. It was concluded that bibliotherapy based on behavioral principles was an effective treatment. Personal contact is not as important as had been traditionally assumed, at least in the treatment of obesity.

Similar results were reported by Hanson (1974) and Bellack, Schwartz, and Rozensky (1974). Hanson (1974) devised a weight reduction manual, using a programmed format. No-treatment control, attention-placebo, and leader-led self-control groups were compared with high- and low-contact bibliotherapy groups. The high-contact group was similar to Hagen's (1974) since the participants met weekly to review the material presented in the programmed text. The low-contact group met briefly with the therapist three times. Measures of percentage of body weight lost and percentage of overweight lost indicated that the three behavioral groups did not differ significantly, but were significantly more effective than either the control or placebo groups. Bellack, Schwartz, and Rozensky (1974) compared three levels of therapist contact in a self-control program. High-contact participants met weekly with the therapist for eight weeks; low-contact participants maintained contact through the mails only; while the no-contact participants had no contact with the therapist between the first and last sessions. Both high- and low-contact groups lost significantly more weight than the no-contact group, although the type of contact did not have any effect on the amount lost.

Jeffrey and Christensen (1972) also found that participants given behavioral instructions and materials, and told to use the procedures on their own, did not lose significantly more weight than a no-treatment control. The results of the above studies seem to indicate that bibliotherapy using behavioral self-control procedures is as effective as a leader-led group using the same procedures. However, some minimal level of therapist contact appears to be necessary.

Exercise Management

Although techniques for increasing energy expenditure have been included as part of several self-control programs (e.g., Stuart 1971), there has been little attempt to investigate experimentally the usefulness of this procedure. On the basis of earlier research which indicated that inactivity is a significant factor in perpetuating obesity, Harris and Hallbauer (1973) hypothesized that a behavioral treatment including exercise would be more effective than a behavioral treatment by itself. They also predicted that both treatments would result in greater weight loss than that obtained by an attention-placebo group. The behavioral treatment common to the two experimental groups included self-control and therapist-reinforcement techniques. There were no significant differences between groups at the end of treatment; however, a seven-month follow-up revealed that the two behavioral groups lost more weight than the attention-placebo group; and the behavioral treatment which included exercise was most successful.

Kau and Fischer (1974) describe a self-modification of exercise program used by the senior author. Her husband dispensed monetary and social reinforcers contingent upon the number of points she earned by jogging. After ten weeks the exercise became intrinsically reinforcing, and the contingencies were no longer necessary.

In view of the demonstrated inactivity of most obese people (Bradfield and Jourdan 1972), exercise management clearly deserves more experimental investigation.

Simple Self-Control

The complex self-control programs, both leader-led and bibliotherapy, make use of a wide variety of techniques and procedures. In addition to the monitoring of food intake, most programs include suggestions for altering the circumstances and patterns of eating, exercise, food shopping, etc. An alternative simple self-control strategy, called "The Mouthful Diet," was proposed by Fowler. Basically, this approach entails counting every mouthful of food and swallow of caloric liquid. Typically, a wrist golf counter is used for this purpose. After a baseline record has been established, the number of mouthfuls per day is systematically decreased in order to produce the desired weight loss. While an increase in the amount of food consumed in each bite is likely to occur, the fixed limit imposed by the size of the mouth will ensure eventual weight reduction as the number of mouthfuls per day is decreased (see chapter 5 for a more complete discussion of this issue).

Fowler et al. (1972) evaluated this approach using sixty-six overweight women. All participants received the same treatment, although there were differences in the method of delivery. Two of the groups met weekly with a therapist for six weeks, while the third group maintained contact by mail. A total of twenty-three participants maintained contact for the full thirty-two-week treatment program. There were no significant differences between treatment groups although personal contact resulted in nonsignificantly greater weight loss. There was, however, a significant difference in weight loss between the twenty-three participants completing treatment and members of a waiting-list control group. Dropouts also lost more than controls, but this difference was not statistically significant.

A second study (Hall et al. 1974) compared a simple self-control program entailing ten brief weekly group meetings with a standard behavioral self-control program, a nonspecific (i.e., group discussion and muscle relaxation), and no-treatment control. At the end of treatment, both self-control procedures resulted in significantly more weight loss than nonspecific or control groups, although there was no significant difference between the self-control groups. Similar results were found at the fourteen-week follow-up, leading the authors to conclude that the simpler procedure is as effective as the complex self-control treatment.

The simplicity of this method lends itself to widespread application. Although there is not yet sufficient evidence to conclude that simple self-control is an effective procedure, the promise of this method warrants additional research.

Coverant Conditioning

Homme (1965) presented a rationale for the reinforcement of thoughts, conceptualized as covert operants (or coverants). This technique entails using highly probable behaviors or thoughts to reinforce low-probability thoughts. Applied to weight control, the low-probability thought (e.g., "if I eat this piece of cake, I will become horribly fat") is reinforced by some high-probability behavior other than eating. Studies reported by Tyler and Straughan (1970) and Horan and Johnson (1971) failed to demonstrate the usefulness of this approach as a treatment for obesity. More recently Brunn and Hedburg (1974) compared group covert reinforcement treatments with placebo treatments. The covert reinforcement treatment consisted of eight one-hour sessions in which the participants were relaxed, instructed to think of scenes in which they avoided unnecessary eating, and then received reinforcement. The experimental treatment was significantly more effective than the control although the average weight loss was less than 3 pounds. Horan et al. (1975) found that positive coverants used to reinforce desirable eating behaviors were significantly more effective than negative coverants which deal with the aversive aspects of being overweight. Even though 75 percent of the participants experiencing the positive coverant treatment lost a minimum of 1 pound per week, the authors, concluded, "At most, coverant control ought to be considered as a highly reactive, albeit short-range, treatment component of a comprehensive program that must also include, for example, stimulus control and dietary information" (p. 71).

Comparison Studies

Several investigators have made outcome studies comparing two or more of the various behavioral treatment strategies. Much of this research has been devoted to comparisons between therapist-reinforcement and complex self-control programs. Harris and Bruner (1971) found that therapist reinforcement resulted in significantly more weight reduction than a self-control treatment, although both treatments produced significant weight losses. A ten-month follow-up demonstrated no appreciable lasting treatment effects for any group. Hall (1972) also found superior results with therapist reinforcement when compared with self-control procedures. This study made use of a single-subject, crossover design in which each participant received five weeks of each treatment. One-half of the subjects received the self-control treatment first, followed by therapist reinforcement, while the order of treatment presentation was reversed for the other subjects. Therapist reinforcement resulted in weight losses averaging 1 pound per week, while the self-control treatment was judged to be relatively ineffectual. A two-year follow-up (Hall 1973) revealed no long-lasting effects of behavioral treatment. Hall cautions against excessive pessimism, however. She feels that the discouraging results may be attributable to a deficiency in the particular program used.

In contrast with the two studies cited above, Jeffrey (1974) found that self-control and therapist reinforcement were equally effective, both treatments producing an average weekly weight loss of approximately 1 pound. A six-week follow-up revealed that subjects in the therapist-reinforcement treatment regained 55 percent of their posttreatment weight loss, while the self-control subjects were able to maintain their weight losses. Jeffrey attributes the success of self-control subjects to an increase in internal orientation (i.e., the belief that an individual can control what happens to him).

Abrahms and Allen (1974) compared the results of a self-control program (using the Stuart and Davis 1972*b* manual) with a combination self-control and therapist-reinforcement treatment. While both were significantly more effective than group pressure or control procedures, no additional benefit resulted from the therapist-reinforcement procedure. In a similar study, Franzini and Grimes (1975) compared Stuart's program with a similar treatment that added contracting. This procedure required that subjects publicly sign a contract which stipulated the desired eating behaviors they would perform. Financial contingencies were not imposed for contract violations. The contract group had a lower attrition rate, but the group using the manual without a contract was more successful in reducing. The authors suggest that the superiority of the no-contract group may have been caused by its higher attrition rate. Unsuccessful subjects dropped out, thereby raising the group average, while unsuccessful subjects in the contract group remained in treatment because of their commitment.

The comparative merits of self-control versus therapist-reinforcement programs remains an unresolved issue. Furthermore, it is likely that the issue will remain clouded until some of the basic methodological problems described in the next section are resolved.

Methodological Issues

Despite the overwhelmingly positive outcomes reported in the studies reviewed, there remain many unresolved issues in the behavioral treatment of obesity. Many of the studies suffer from methodological difficulties which limit the generalizability of their results. In interpreting the findings, it is necessary to differentiate between statistical significance and clinical utility. The typical study reports a statistically significant difference between the weight lost by the control group and the weight losses of the treatment groups. The average weight loss of the experimental groups, however, may have been a few pounds. This type of finding is important to the researcher trying to develop a new technique or isolate the potent components of currently available techniques, but it may have limited usefulness to the clinician who is confronted with a grossly overweight client.

Comparison of the results of outcome studies is difficult because of different methods of reporting results (Bellack and Rozensky 1975). Investigators have been interested in the weight losses of their subjects. Despite the ease of measuring weight changes, there is no agreed-upon convention for reporting results. Thus investigators have reported average number of pounds lost, average reductions in percent overweight, and percent of a treatment group reaching or exceeding an arbitrarily defined criterion (e.g., weight loss of 20 pounds or more). The net effect is to make comparisons between studies difficult. Adoption of a Weight Reduction Index which takes into account weight, height, number of pounds overweight, target weight, and pounds lost has been advocated by Jeffrey (1975a). This index, first proposed by Feinstein (1959) is computed as follows:

$$WRI = (W_l/W_s)\,(W_i/W_t) \times 100$$

where: W_l = weight loss; W_s = surplus weight
         W_i = initial weight; W_t = target weight

Franzini and Grimes (1976a) propose that the measurement of weight be abandoned in favor of skinfold measures. They point out that measures of skinfold thickness at the triceps muscle can be easily transformed to a percentage of body fat. They feel that this would be appropriate since obesity is usually viewed as an excessive accumulation of fat. The adoption of this or any standardized index would allow for comparison of different treatments in different studies. Until a standard index is widely used, it would be helpful if investigators reported the beginning and final weights of their subjects.

An additional difficulty in comparing the effects of various behavioral treatment programs is the lack of consistency in reporting data from subjects who drop out of treatment before completion. It seems reasonable to assume that the majority of dropouts were not losing weight and became discouraged. Many of the studies reviewed do not describe any attempt to contact these subjects to find out their weight at the end of the treatment period. This practice has the effect of inflating the average weight loss for the group and makes comparison with other studies that include this data difficult.

Perhaps the most critical methodological shortcoming in most of the research is the lack of long-term follow-ups. As a result of the practical difficulties in locating subjects months or years after participation in treatment, the typical study makes use of a single follow-up between six weeks and three months after completion of treatment. When longer periods are used (e.g., S.M. Hall 1973), the results tend to be disappointing. Stuart's (1967) early case report suggests that occasional maintenance sessions may be useful. He provided them as needed for the eight women he treated, all of whom continued to lose weight. The wide range of treatments required during the course of a year (between sixteen and forty-one) suggests that there may be individual differences in the need for continued therapist contact. In an experimental test, R.G. Hall (1974) found that continued monitoring by mail was as effective as booster sessions with the original therapist and more effective than booster sessions with a new therapist. The obvious implication of these studies is that some form of continued contact will increase the likelihood of maintenance or continued weight losses. Further research will be required to determine the maximally effective format for continued contact. It is not premature, however, to include booster sessions routinely in all weight control programs.

Future Research

Several major questions about behavioral programs remain unanswered. Mahoney (1975*a*) has pointed out that there is no evidence demonstrating that obese individuals participating in self-control programs actually make use of the various techniques that comprise the program. The studies demonstrate that the experimental subjects lose more weight than the controls. This finding suggests but does not prove that the experimental subjects made use of all or some of the suggested techniques. Chlouverakis (1975) reports anecdotally that the more sophisticated of his patients find the various techniques childish and presumably lose interest in them. Additional research will be required to determine patterns of use and attitudes toward the various techniques.

In the research literature, some treatments use a group format while others involve individual sessions with the therapist. Similarly, several investigators have made use of brief sessions that take place two or more times per week while others make use of the traditional fifty-minute hour. The relative effectiveness of the various formats has not been investigated.

Several of the more commonly used self-control techniques (e.g., putting utensils down after each bite in order to increase the duration of eating) are based on questionable assumptions about the eating patterns of the obese. Mahoney (1975*b*) and Gaul, Craighead, and Mahoney (1975) report the results of several laboratory and field studies which failed to support the assumption that obese and nonobese individuals differ in eating style. These findings suggest that it may be possible to streamline the self-control programs by deleting procedures based on fallacious assumptions.

Many of the studies reviewed have included some attempt to

predict, typically on the basis of demographic variables or psychological test scores, which of the subjects would benefit from treatment. If successful, this would allow the therapist to screen potential patients. Ultimately, this strategy would enable differing subtypes of obese individuals to be matched with specific treatments. Unfortunately, little success has been reported. Variables which have been unsuccessful in predicting treatment outcome include the following: extraversion-introversion, general anxiety, situational anxiety, physical activity, self-reports of frequency of various eating behaviors (Wollersheim 1970), the Minnesota Multiphasic Personality Inventory, and Maudsley Personality Inventory (Jeffrey, Christensen, and Pappas 1972). Results with the Internal-External Locus of Control Inventory have been conflicting. Jeffrey, Christensen, and Pappas (1972) were unsuccessful in predicting treatment outcome while Balch and Ross (1975) reported significant correlations between I-E scores and weight loss.

Borden (1974) found that socioeconomic status was positively related to the number of pounds lost (i.e., higher-status subjects lost more weight). Also, participants who were older when they first became obese were more successful during and after treatment. Other findings included a negative correlation between pounds lost and number of previous attempts to lose weight. The number of medical problems reported and number of reasons for wanting to lose weight were positively related to success in treatment. A recent attempt to devise a regression equation that would predict success in behavioral treatment was unsuccessful (Henley 1976). The variables used to make the predictions were deduced from both Schachter's and Nisbett's theories. The most encouraging finding was reported by Bellack (1975). A self-reinforcement task was administered to subjects undergoing behavioral treatment. Subjects who tended to be more self-reinforcing lost more weight than those who were less likely to reinforce themselves. If this finding is replicated, it may become possible to identify those individuals who are most likely to benefit from behavioral treatment.

Etiology and Treatment

A basic, and unresolved, issue is the degree to which biological factors limit the applicability and success of behavioral treatments. Whatever the underlying biological factors, there is a consensus that obese individuals suffer from a positive energy balance (i.e., they consume more calories than they need).

The biological factors manifest themselves in the overt behaviors of excessive food consumption and/or inadequate exercise. These overt behaviors are subject to the same types of environmental control as other overt behaviors. Stunkard (1975) reviewed the literature dealing with social and cultural factors in obesity and concluded "whatever its genetic determinants and its biochemical pathways, obesity is to an unusual degree under social environmental control" (p. 207). He suggested that treatment of obesity is not dependent upon complete understanding of its biochemical determinants; an understanding of the social factors may suffice.

Assuming that Stunkard's position is correct, behavioral researchers and therapists, nonetheless, should be aware of the influences of biological factors on the course of treatment. The individual's age at onset of obesity may be a critical variable. Early onset obesity, resulting from genetic and/or excessive caloric intake during critical periods in infancy, results in a larger number of fat cells which remains constant throughout life. Adult onset obesity results in the increase in size of the fat cells while the number of cells remains constant. Reduction for the juvenile onset obese may be more difficult since it requires the "starvation" of fat cells. Research has demonstrated that the juvenile onset obese experience anxiety, depression, and preoccupation with food during weight reduction. The adult onset obese, on the other hand, display little emotional disturbance while reducing (Glucksman and Hirsch 1968; Glucksman et al. 1968; Grinker, Hirsch, and Levin 1973). The obvious implication for behavioral treatment is that reduction will be more difficult for juvenile onset patients. Borden's (1974) findings, cited above, are consistent with this hypothesis. At present there has been no attempt to deal with this problem. Behavior therapists may have to expand their treatment packages to include techniques aimed at alleviating the discomfort that results from weight loss. These might be included in the booster sessions previously described.

In summary, it is important that the reader recognize the tentative nature of the procedures described in the programs presented in this book. There are many unresolved issues in the behavioral treatment of obesity. It is inevitable that the treatments will be modified in light of new research findings. The reader is encouraged to keep informed about new developments.

part II

behavioral treatment programs

The readings in this section provide the information necessary to conduct a behavioral self-control program. Chapters 3 and 4 describe the format and specific techniques required for a complex self-control treatment while chapter 5 relates the procedures involved in simple self-control. These treatment manuals should not be considered sacred. After reviewing the research findings presented in chapter 2, and the clinical issues discussed in chapter 9, the reader may decide to modify the program to fit the specific needs of the population to be treated. For example, one or more of the techniques presented in part III could be added. In light of the considerable variation in the content of the self-control programs used by experimenters, it is unlikely that minor modifications will do any damage. Radical alteration, on the other hand, may result in a program that lacks the experimental validation of the original.

Christensen, Jeffrey, and Pappas (chapter 3) present detailed instructions for arranging and conducting a self-control program. The program is divided into four phases which include both individual and group meetings. This is a worthwhile feature since it allows the economies of group treatment while still providing for the individualization of treatment. Several other features merit comment. The Intake Phase of the program is intended to determine the prospective group member's suitability for treatment. The interview, along with the Weight Reduction Program Questionnaire (appendix A), allows the therapist to plan for individual difficulties that may interfere with treatment. When these difficulties make it unlikely that treatment will succeed, the therapist may suggest that the patient seek counseling or psychotherapy to resolve the problem prior to starting treatment.

The authors suggest that the first two weeks of treatment be devoted to a Baseline Phase. This period is devoted to building group cohesion and establishing a pretreatment measure of calorie consumption. Since many of the group members will be eager to begin treatment, it may be advisable to combine the Baseline and Standardized Treatment Phases, especially since self-monitoring is frequently a treatment (i.e., it results in weight loss). Another feature of the program which can be questioned is the requirement that participants weigh themselves daily. Mahoney and Mahoney (1976b) suggest that daily weight checks can have a destructive influence on the participant's morale. In my weight control groups I have encouraged weekly rather than daily weigh-ins. Although many patients find it difficult to discontinue their daily (sometimes hourly!) checking, the net effect is to reduce the inevitable discouragement that occurs when a day of reduced caloric consumption is not followed by a noticeable weight loss.

The appendixes for chapter 3 can be found at the end of the book and include a variety of forms which would be useful for any of the behavioral treatments along with several case histories illustrating behavioral treatment. The case histories demonstrate the role of nonspecific influences on treatment outcome and thereby emphasize the need for sensitivity on the part of the therapist conducting the treatment. While the authors suggest one technique for increasing group cohesiveness at the start of the program, this may be insufficient. Readers lacking previous experience with therapeutic groups would profit from a text on group leadership (e.g., Bates and Johnson 1972).

In chapter 4 Wollersheim describes the various techniques that make up the contents of a complex self-control program. This material can be used in two ways: the therapist can present and lead discussions of the various techniques during the Standardized and Individualized Treatment Phases of the program described in chapter 3, or, the material can be rewritten for use as a bibliotherapy manual tailored to the needs of a specified treatment group. Hagen's (1974) successful bibliotherapy was based largely on this manual.

Chapter 4 was taken from a treatment manual used to train group leaders for a weight reduction study conducted with college women (hence the use of feminine pronouns). This manual is probably the most comprehensive list of self-control techniques currently available. Since there is considerable variation between participants in the effectiveness of any one technique, Wollersheim suggests that the therapist should encourage each group member to try each technique for at least one week. Although comprehensive, this chapter does not include all of the possible techniques for self-control. The therapist and group members may devise additional applications or variations of the techniques presented in order to meet specific needs.

The therapist planning on using Wollersheim's techniques as part of the program presented in chapter 3 may want to change the order in which the

techniques are presented. For example, "Keeping records of eating behavior" (i.e., self-monitoring)
should probably be the first technique introduced.
Also, Wollersheim suggests a weekly weight loss goal
of 2 pounds. While this is entirely appropriate for
college students, middle-aged women may not be
able to accomplish this without excessively reducing
their caloric intake. A weekly goal of 1 pound or
even ½ pound may be more appropriate for some
participants.

In chapter 5 Fowler presents a simple self-control program which he calls "The Mouthful Diet." It
is written as a self-help manual suitable for use with
minimal therapist contact. The therapist planning on
using this program should be aware of several concerns. First, simple self-control has not been evaluated as extensively as complex self-control. The
available research suggests that it is as effective as
the more complex programs, but it would be premature to draw definitive conclusions. A second potential concern is that the program deals exclusively
with eating. There are some individuals who become
obese as a result of a sedentary life-style even though
they do not eat excessvely. It is unlikely that simple
self-control would benefit these people. Finally, the
therapist should be prepared to encounter some re-
sistance to the use of a golf counter to measure food
consumption. Many, if not most, obese individuals
are self-conscious about anything relating to eating.
It is unlikely, therefore, that they will be eager to use
the golf counter in public since this would draw attention to their obvious weight problem.

In summary, chapter 3 presents the basic format
for a complex self-control program. Chapter 4 describes the specific techniques that will be taught to
the participants in the program. This combination
would be the preferred treatment for most applications. The therapist recognizing its experimental nature may want to use the program presented in
chapter 5 because of its simplicity.

③

A Therapist Manual for a Behavior Modification Weight Reduction Program

Edwin R. Christensen, D. Balfour Jeffrey, and James P. Pappas

This outpatient behavior modification program was developed in order to provide services for the common problem of obesity. References for the techniques used in this program and demonstrations of its effectiveness are included elsewhere (Jeffrey 1973; Jeffrey and Christensen 1972; Jeffrey, Christensen, and Pappas 1972). There are also a number of other studies that have appeared in recent years which support the behavioral therapy approach to obesity (see Stunkard 1972).

This manual's purpose is to provide information and suggestions which will facilitate implementation of this approach in an agency. It is intended for use by professionals skilled in working

This chapter was originally published as Research and Development Report No. 37, Counseling and Psychological Services, University of Utah. Copyright © 1973 by the authors. All Rights Reserved. Used with permission.

The authors wish to thank all the clients who have participated in our weight program and who have given us helpful information on how to improve the program. The authors would also like to thank the Counseling and Psychological Services, in particular Dr. Ted Packard and the secretarial staff, for their continuous support.

47

with people. The program is developed for use in either a group or
an individual setting. An overview of each phase of the program is
presented first.

Intake

During the intake interview, the therapist assesses the patient's
present commitment to losing weight, his weight history, and general life situation.

Initial or Baseline Phase

In the initial group meeting, the therapist-group leader explains
the program and instructs patients not to lose weight the first two
weeks. He also explains that there is one 45-minute and one
5-minute meeting for patients to attend each week. He tells them to
monitor daily weight and to write down everything they eat during
the week. This is done so that baseline or pretreatment data can be
obtained. From these data the group leader assesses group members'
caloric intake patterns.

Standardized Treatment Phase

At the first meeting of this phase, the group leader explains and
implements the response-cost procedure. A sum of money deposited
with the therapist is to be used as reinforcement for the self-monitoring procedures, attendance and weight loss. When a weekly
weight loss goal is attained by a patient, a portion of the deposit will
be returned. However, when the weight loss goal is not attained, a
portion of the deposit will be lost. In essence, if the eating response
is too great during the week, then it "costs" the individual the potential reinforcement. The therapist will use the same procedure for
shaping the patient's self-monitoring and attendance.

The therapist-group leader then instructs the patients to develop an energy expenditure program, which is any form of physical
exercise, such as walking instead of driving to work. He also gives
the group members specific stimulus control procedures to follow,
such as leaving all food in the kitchen. The verbal statements and
comments of the therapist and other group members are to be used
as reinforcers for these portions of the program.

Also during this phase, patients write down the negative consequences of not losing weight and the positive consequences of losing weight. The group leader then gives instructions to read these statements during the weigh-in sessions and before meals.

Group members write all of these procedures, along with the reinforcements contingent on their accomplishment or nonaccomplishment, in a document called a contingency contract. Both the group members and group leader sign the contract.

As this phase of the program continues, individual patients' proclivities and difficulties appear. As a result, the individualized phase of the program is progressively instituted.

Individualized Treatment Phase

The therapist and group members gradually tailor treatment procedures to fit individuals. For example, instead of using monetary reinforcement, a patient could report progress in specific terms to other group members and then receive praise or other social-verbal reinforcement from the group leader and group members.

During this phase, the group leader institutes reinforcement-thinning and stimulus-fading. He does this by changing the weekly 5-minute weigh-in to a phone call and then finally terminating it altogether. Next, he changes the weekly 45-minute sessions, where reinforcement and discussion of problems occur, to biweekly sessions. In this way, the therapist-controlled reinforcements and stimuli are gradually thinned and faded so that control for weight loss or maintenance of the loss is shifted to the patient. As the final weight goal is achieved, individual group members begin the next phase.

Maintenance Follow-up Phase

The purpose of this phase is to test the permanence of the change in eating habits. The patient and the therapist negotiate meeting times and dates for the maintenance period. The meetings are sometimes conducted individually, with the therapist's verbal comments serving as the main source of reinforcement.

Each of these phases will be explained in greater detail in the following sections of the manual. The examples used come from patient histories. For additional case histories illustrating various aspects of the program, refer to appendix I.

Intake

The system used for intake of patients need not be altered from any standard system used in the therapist's agency. However, it is profitable to be sensitive to some unique cues which are pertinent in assessing and treating obesity. A weight reduction questionnaire can be helpful in providing information on some of these cues (see appendix A).

Behavioral, Psychological, and Physical Difficulties Which May Hinder Weight Reduction Treatment

Certain difficulties of patients may interfere with success in a weight reduction program. For example, someone who experiences anxiety from heterosexual interaction may become more anxious as weight is lost because of a "fear" of becoming attractive to the opposite sex. Other individuals may find it difficult to lose weight because eating is associated with reduction of anxiety over difficulties such as familial discord, poor academic performance, or other problems. Or a middle-aged man, who may have a desire to be young and slim-looking, may be on a high caloric diet for stomach ulcers. If these or other difficulties exist, multiple or alternate interventions may be appropriate (see appendix I, case 1). Where multiple interventions are needed because of other psychological difficulties, it is generally more effective to have a separate therapist for weight reduction treatment.

Patient Difficulties Which May Aid in Weight Reduction

Some concerns may aid in weight reduction treatment by providing a stimulus for making a commitment, such as a genuine desire to be more attractive to the opposite sex, or to decrease the risk of heart failure. An occasional reminder of such concerns during treatment can be helpful. These cues can also be included in a "reinforcement menu" and then used formally as a reinforcement (see appendix E).

Other Treatments

Past or present performance in other programs for weight reduction can give information as to how committed a patient is to losing weight and maintaining loss. If a person has been unsuccessful in other programs, greater magnitude and/or density of reinforcement than usual may be necessary. Or, if he has been successful at losing weight but not at maintaining the loss, greater attention may need to be given to contingencies in the maintenance phase of this program. Treatments for individuals with diabetes, ulcers, heart conditions, and other physical ailments will require consultation with a physician.

Also, past or present treatments for other difficulties of a psychological nature are indicators of variables which may influence weight reduction treatment, as already mentioned.

Weight History and Goals

The length of time a patient has been overweight is useful information which may indicate how much difficulty he will have making weekly loss goals. Experience suggests that if the gain is recent, generally the loss will be easier; if it is chronic, the loss will be more difficult.

The weight that a patient wishes to attain is useful information. It gives the therapist an indication of how long the loss will take, how much has to be lost, and if the desired weight is realistic. Also, present weight should be measured on an accurate scale so that the therapist has a pretreatment measure of weight.

Commitment to Losing Weight

An assessment of the patient's commitment to losing weight should be obtained. Four questions have proven helpful in this assessment and also aid in helping the patient to respond to the issue:

1. Will the effort be worth the payoff?
2. Why does he desire to lose weight?
3. What is he willing to sacrifice to lose weight?
4. Will his spouse and friends help or hinder his commitment to lose weight?

These questions are not all that may be pertinent but are a minimum for use in assessing and treating obesity. As an additional aid, all or portions of the *Outline of Interview Information Needed for a Functional Analysis* may be helpful (Kanfer and Saslow 1965).

Initial or Baseline Phase: Explaining the Program and Implementing Baseline Procedures

In the first session the group leader gives an overview of the program. He should explain that this program is designed to help a patient reduce to his weight goal and then maintain that weight by doing the following: (1) conditioning a change in eating habits, (2) earning rewards contingent on reaching weekly loss goals, attending therapy sessions, doing the necessary tasks (such as cutting caloric intake, graphing daily weight, and instituting the stimulus control instructions), and attaining the final desired weight.

The group leader can then give more detail by going through a standardized contract item by item and explaining briefly what each means (see appendix B).

If the program is being conducted using a group format, the group leader should attempt to build group cohesion by any methods he knows. One method to develop surface familiarity is to allow five minutes for pairs of patients to get to know something about each other and then to introduce their partner to the group.

Next, the group should establish the meeting times for each week. This is done so that there is a 45-minute session and an additional 5-minute weigh-in session each week.

Patients are given eating diaries in which items and amounts eaten are to be recorded until the next week's session (see appendix G). Patients are also given a daily weight graph. At this time the contracts are not yet filled out, but encouragement should be given to have final weight goals in mind. Instructions should also be given for each individual to bring a physician's statement concerning his physical condition.

At the second session the group leader asks each patient to bring money or objects for deposit by the next week so that they can be used as reinforcers the following week. The deposit should be large enough so that the amount earned back weekly will be significantly reinforcing. Instructions are given on how to count average daily caloric intake for each of six eating time periods representing meals and snacks following meals (for computing instructions, see appendix H). Also, physicians' statements should be collected. An outline of the initial or baseline sessions follows:

FIRST 45-MINUTE SESSION:

1. The patients weigh in.

2. An overview and explanation of the program is given.

3. Introductions and initial attempts at building group cohesion are instituted.

4. Eating diaries and weight graphs are given out.

5. Physicians' statement forms are handed out (due by the following week).

SECOND 45-MINUTE SESSION:

1. The patients weigh in.

2. The therapist states that reinforcement deposits are due by next week.

3. Physicians' statements are collected.

4. Eating diaries are collected, and preliminary assessment of caloric intake patterns are made.

5. Daily weight graphs are examined by the group leader.

6. Instructions on how to compute and analyze daily and weekly caloric intake patterns are given.

Later in the week, a 5-minute individual meeting should also be conducted at which the patient merely weighs in and shows his weight graphs to the therapist.

During the baseline sessions, shaping also occurs so that the following behaviors are conditioned:

1. Daily weigh-in at home,

2. Recording daily weight on graphs,

3. Attendance at both weekly meetings.

During this initial or baseline phase, patients are often made so aware of how much they eat that they will begin to lose weight. The therapist may verbally reinforce this loss but not with formal monetary contingencies until the next phase of the program is begun.

Standardized Treatment Phase

In the first treatment session the group members establish their final desired-weight goal. Often the tendency is to set this goal too high. Some middle-aged patients will try to establish their desired weight at what it was when they were in high school, which is probably not realistic. To avoid this, interim goals can be instituted for any desired weight loss exceeding 20 pounds. After the first 20 pounds are lost, a new goal can be set. Experience suggests that setting goals too far from the present weight can be discouraging, seemingly unattainable, and may become a negative stimulus for weight loss. Contingencies may or may not be established for the attainment of the final weight goal, depending on individual preferences. Cash rewards or objects of value may be deposited so that they may be obtained when the goal is reached.

Patients should next set the weekly weight loss goal to which response-cost contingencies will be applied in each 45-minute weekly session. It is important that the goals set encourage a gradual weight loss. Sudden losses are not usually accompanied by permanent changes in eating habits; thus, the loss is not maintained. A weekly loss falling between 1 and 2 pounds is usually the most appropriate. Individuals who are very obese will often be able to lose more weight per week initially than individuals who are moderately obese.

The patient's reinforcement deposit will be used in the weekly response-cost procedure. Initially neither patient nor therapist knows how much weekly reinforcement or loss of reinforcement in monetary terms will be enough to condition weight loss behavior. For students with small incomes, amounts earned from their deposits may initially vary between $2 and $10 per week. For someone working full time, larger amounts may be more appropriate. For some, to earn physical objects which have been deposited has more reinforcement value. The objects should be amenable to being earned piecemeal. Record collections, golf clubs, favorite books, and favorite items of clothing are examples of objects which may be deposited with the therapist. In addition to being used for weekly reinforcements, these and other objects can also be used as reinforcement when the final weight goal is attained.

A "dropout" contingency should also be negotiated. One

method would be to have the patient lose all money or objects deposited if he drops out before attaining his goal.

If enough time remains in the first treatment session, goals concerning altering eating habits and instituting stimulus control procedures can be put on the contract. If enough time does not remain, they can be put in the following session.

The necessary alterations in patients' patterns of timing and amount of caloric intake can be suggested from data on the eating diary. For example, patients often eat very little in the morning and very heavily in the evenings. To increase caloric intake in the morning and greatly reduce it in the evening may be appropriate instead of merely reducing the caloric intake in the evening. Other patterns may show one specific time of high caloric intake and the need to reduce the intake drastically at that time while maintaining the same caloric intake level at other times. Another pattern may be a fairly high caloric intake between meals. To lower intake significantly at these times may reduce the total intake sufficiently. As a general rule, fairly significant caloric intake reductions are needed in order to lose weight. A reduction of approximately 3,500 calories is needed for a 1-pound weight loss. Additionally, if more calories are "burned" through energy expenditure procedures, the patients' weight loss and muscle tone will be improved (see appendix I, case 5).

Stimulus control procedures wherein the clients institute specific changes in their eating habits have been previously developed (Ferster, Nurnberger, and Levitt 1961; Mahoney and Jeffrey 1973; Stuart 1967, 1971). These techniques should be instituted by each client at the pace of about one per week. An outline of these procedures follows, and a separate booklet has been written to give each client (Mahoney and Jeffrey 1973). The booklet includes specific techniques for weight control, procedures on how to record one's weight and eating habits, and some basic facts about nutrition.

Specific Weight Control Techniques

The weight control techniques are divided into the following three categories: *quantity control,* referring to how much is eaten; *quality control,* referring to what is eaten; and *situation control,* referring to where and when one eats. The following headings are quotations from Mahoney and Jeffrey (1973).

QUANTITY CONTROL TECHNIQUES:

1. Reduce the amount of food you prepare and serve.
2. Leave food on your plate.
3. Eat slowly.

QUALITY CONTROL TECHNIQUES:

1. Keep a supply of dietetic or unfattening foods on hand.
2. Avoid high caloric snacks.
3. Do not adorn fattening foods.

SITUATION CONTROL TECHNIQUES:

1. Separate eating from all other activities.
2. Eat only if you are hungry.
3. Delay your gratification.
4. Restrict yourself before you eat.
5. Buy and prepare food on a full stomach.
6. Enlist the help of your loved ones and friends.

The stimulus control procedures should be discussed, verbally reinforced, and progressively instituted at each succeeding group meeting after the initial standardized treatment meeting. A summary of the first 45-minute standardized treatment meeting is given below. (As the following are accomplished, the patient should fill in the contingency contract.)

1. Group members weigh in.
2. Final desired weight goal and reinforcements for its attainment are set.
3. Weekly weight loss goals are set.
4. Reinforcement deposits are collected.
5. Portions of the patients' deposits to be used for weekly reinforcement are set.
6. A dropout contingency is negotiated.
7. Final assessments of caloric intake patterns are made from the eating diary.
8. If time remains, goals are set for altering caloric intake patterns, reducing caloric intake, instituting energy expenditure procedures, and instituting stimulus control procedures. (If

time does not remain, these can be accomplished the following session.)

9. The contingency contracts are signed by both the patients and the therapist.

In the succeeding sessions during this phase, the following week's weight goal should be clearly indicated on both the patient's and the therapist's copies of the daily weight graph and verbally stated. Also, the contingency on the weekly weight loss should be clearly stated and understood by both parties. Reminders of both the goal and contingencies on its attainment should be given at the 5-minute weigh-in session.

What usually takes place during the two weekly sessions follows.

45-MINUTE SESSION. (As final goals come nearer to being reached, reinforcement-thinning and stimulus-fading become appropriate, which can be accomplished by changing from weekly to biweekly meetings and finally by their termination.)

1. Patients weigh in.
2. Therapist transcribes daily weights from patients' graphs to his copy.
3. Next week's goal is indicated on the graph (appendix C).
4. Monetary rewards are given in the group for attendance at both meetings during the week and for weight loss.
5. Progress in instituting stimulus control procedures, in following energy expenditure programs, in lowering caloric intake, and in altering eating patterns are discussed and verbally reinforced. (Note: By the therapist's spending a great deal of attention and/or time on one individual's failure, the patient may be reinforced for no weight loss or no change in eating habits. If this is a consistent pattern, a confrontation and recommitment to weight loss, while ignoring the previous attention-getting behavior, would be more appropriate. Confrontation can be talking about commitment or showing the patient his *weekly* weight graph, in addition to other confrontive behaviors found effective by the therapist.)

5-MINUTE WEIGH-IN SESSION. (As final goals are nearer to being reached, reinforcement-thinning and stimulus-fading become appropriate, which can be accomplished by changing this meeting to a phone call and later terminating it altogether.)

1. Patient weighs in.
2. Group leader transcribes weight from the patient's graph to his copy.
3. Group leader gives a reminder of next week's weight goal and how much weight has to be lost by the upcoming 45-minute session.
4. Verbal reinforcements are given, but no monetary reinforcements are given unless individually contracted.

Individualized Treatment Phase

A shift to more individualized treatment occurs as the therapist and patient observe and respond to the following:

1. Total weight loss since the beginning of the program.
2. The *weekly* weight loss as recorded on the therapist's *weekly* weight loss graph (see appendix D).
3. Attendance, daily graphing, and the accomplishment of the other tasks.
4. What is and is not most reinforcing for the individual. (Careful observation, questions, and responses to the reinforcement menus are helpful in this assessment.)
5. The effect of different amounts and timing of reinforcement.
6. Which stimulus control procedures seem to be most effective.

Experimentation, assessment, and altering of different aspects of the program should occur in order to maximize weight loss. As a result, a gradual restructuring of each patient's treatment program should also occur. Increased or decreased weekly goals may be desirable, or alternative structuring of weekly weight goals may become appropriate. One alternative method is to negotiate the amount of weight to be lost for the following week at each 45-minute weekly session. This may be helpful if someone has lost weight in widely varying amounts because of intervening environmental factors. For example, a woman may be able to lose more during some weeks and less during others because of water-weight gain at certain times in her menstrual cycle. Another method of scheduling weekly goals is to draw a downward slanting line on the weight graphs with the contingencies centering at or below the line for each weekly weigh-in. This can be effective where a sawtooth up and down pattern is apparent with little mean weight loss. However, caution should be used with this method. If the required weight loss is not attained in the first week or two and continues not to be attained, failure to meet goals may become regular. This tendency can partially be controlled by not making the slope of the line more than an individual has demonstrated he can lose during weekly intervals in the past. Also, a definite recommitment with a larger deposit, so that there is greater magnitude of reinforcement, will help condition consistent weekly weight loss.

Some people have difficulty controlling their caloric intake on weekends. If this occurs, the two group meeting times can be changed to Fridays and Mondays. This will aid in the control of caloric intake during the intervening period. If this cannot be done, then the patient can phone the therapist on Fridays and Mondays to make goals and receive verbal reinforcement for achieving the goals.

When patients are not doing well, they get discouraged and occasionally wish to drop out. When this happens, the therapist should remind the patient of his goals and the positive consequences of achieving these goals. Encouraging remarks and frequent presentation of the patient's progress since the beginning of the program can be reinforcing. Also, it can be important to use persuasive behavior and encouragement to get the patient to recommit himself to the idea of losing weight. The potential side effects of dropping out and/or perceived failure by the patient may make it important for him to keep with his goal to lose weight.

During this portion of the program, assessment may also show that a change in the nature of reinforcement is necessary. Some patients may respond to monetary reinforcers best (see appendix I, case 3), but others may respond better to different kinds of reinforcers. For example, the actual weight loss may be viewed as most reinforcing, with monetary payments viewed as bribery. If this happens, the monetary reinforcers may be dropped, and concentration on the weekly graph and social reinforcers may be more appropriate.

With some individuals, stimulus materials or objects are useful as reminders, such as statements of consequences for losing or not losing weight (see appendix E). Also, photographs or small toys have been used as stimuli to remind patients of their commitments (see appendix I, case 6). Where, when, and how these objects will be displayed can be written into contracts. For example, a contract might specify that a photograph showing the patient as overweight be displayed on the refrigerator door, or that the individual read his statements of consequences before meals. Generally, effective use of stimulus objects occurs as individual programs become more tailor-made.

As the desired weight is attained, the next phase of the program is begun.

Maintenance Follow-up Phase

This phase is perhaps the most important because it is when the permanence of eating behavior changes and the patient's control are tested. It is, therefore, important that follow-up and/or maintenance sessions be conducted.

The procedures used here are essentially extensions of the individualized treatment phase with significantly reduced frequency of meetings. The monetary contingencies are dropped unless requests are made for booster sessions and it seems that these contingencies need to be reinstated (see appendix I, case 4). The resetting of goals, recommitment, and social-verbal reinforcement are generally all that are necessary. The spacing and timing of sessions during this phase are individually determined. Some groups desire to meet together; others do not. Some individuals may desire meeting more or less often than others. It is probably best to set dates and times when the sessions will be held before this phase is begun so that there is precommitment to meet after long lapses of time.

A way to set maintenance goals during this phase is to draw a horizontal line across the weight graphs at the point below which the client desires to stay and then to base reinforcement on whether or not the weight is above or below this line. Commitments should be obtained in the same manner for this phase as for the earlier phases.

Therapist Behaviors

Certain therapist behaviors facilitate the treatment program.

One facilitative behavior is for the therapist to give verbal reinforcement which is viewed as positive. This does not always mean direct approval or encouragement. Some individuals may view approval and/or encouragement negatively. Others may view it as neither positive nor negative. Still others may view it positively. Therapists should experiment and make assessments in order to find what is or is not reinforcing to each individual.

Another set of behaviors found to be effective in this program is to be direct and candid in presenting what a patient's performance has been, or is at present. Visual presentation of daily and weekly weight graphs with an accompanying explanation is a good example of such behavior. Any pointing out of successes or failures in performance, if well timed and presented, is reinforcing in most cases.

The therapist should be aware of the importance of the potential social reinforcement available in the weight reduction group. In order to take advantage of this potential, he should encourage all goals, problems, and progress being made public to the other group members. He should also encourage group members to contribute reinforcing comments, etc., to other group members concerning their progress. Reinforcements from the group to an individual are probably a significant factor in successful treatment.

Sensitivity to competing variables is important. Patients will sometimes be reinforced from unknown sources. Competing reinforcements can be more powerful than those the therapist might impose (see appendix I, case 2). For example, one weight therapist was seeing together two patients who were friends. As time went on, neither of the two was losing a significant amount of weight. Alerted by verbal cues, the therapist questioned the two friends about the possibility of reinforcing each other to indulge in high caloric intake. This proved to be what was happening. Seeing them separately and verbally committing each to reinforce the other to lower caloric intake alleviated the difficulty.

The setting of goals is an important part of this program. The therapist should be a negotiator in this process. In any negotiation the individual is neither told what his goals should be nor allowed to set goals which would be too difficult to obtain. Often the initial goals tend to be set too high, and there will be a need to make interim goals or to renegotiate the goals later. It is facilitative to allow renegotiations of goals where it is evident that keeping present unattainable goals would condition failure in the program.

Another important set of behaviors for the therapist is to be constantly up to date with his graphs and other assessments of a patient's progress so that he can be sensitive to any changes in behavior or environment which might alter performance.

In summary, it is important for the environment to be such that patients can emit correct behaviors, and it is equally important that therapists emit behaviors that create such an environment.

4

Behavioral Techniques for Weight Control

Janet P. Wollersheim

This chapter describes and explains the specific therapeutic techniques to be used in the learning theory treatment for helping participants change their eating patterns so that they will lose weight. Once they reach their desired weight, they will have developed "normal" eating habits appropriate to maintaining their weight at this level. The techniques are described in the order in which they are to be introduced and implemented in the discussion phases of the separate therapy sessions. It is emphasized that, while these techniques have been designed to be maximally effective in aiding individuals to modify their eating behavior and consequently lose weight, they must be *applied* and *used* by individual members. Discussion alone will not bring about desirable results. *The therapist's most important task is to help each individual specifically implement these techniques in a manner appropriate to the circumstances and situations arising in her particular mode of living.*

This chapter was adapted with minor modifications from *Therapist treatment manual for the Focal Therapy based on learning principles* (available through *JSAS Catalog of Selected Documents in Psychology*). Used with permission.

When the techniques are first introduced, the therapist must take care to explain them well, defining and explaining terms as the need arises and eliciting feedback from the group to ensure that they understand precisely the way in which the technique must be implemented in order to be effective. Discussion should be elicited from the participants concerning the manner in which each member can implement the technique in her living pattern. The first half of the discussion phase in the session is to be spent checking on how each member has been implementing the techniques, with more attention devoted to the techniques introduced in the previous session but with routine checking of all techniques introduced to that point. Misunderstandings and errors in application are to be corrected during the discussion phase with the therapist himself providing support, encouragement, reinforcement, and persuasion as well as eliciting these from the group.

It is to be expected that not all individuals will find all techniques equally effective, nor will individuals be equally disposed to implement and apply all techniques to the same degree. The therapist is to encourage participants to try all techniques at least for the week following their initial introduction, and then he can explain that the members can focus more upon those techniques which they have found most effective and which seem to be more applicable to their individual eating habits. However, should the patient be omitting a technique that would seem very important in helping her acquire more appropriate eating habits, the therapist must call this to her attention and try to persuade and encourage her to utilize the particular procedure.

In the course of treatment, participants may introduce ideas relating to techniques not yet formally introduced. When this occurs, instructions concerning the technique should be given to ensure that the participants will be applying it correctly. However, the technique is again to be explained and discussed in the session designated for this. If a participant introduces a worthwhile technique not formally included in the treatment outline, it can be discussed if it seems to be of value to the individual. Again the purpose of the discussion would be to aid the participant in proper application. Techniques which participants introduce and which are poorly adapted to promoting appropriate eating habits should be identified as such, accompanied by an explanation of why they are likely to be ineffective.

An explanation of the techniques used in this treatment condition follows. The therapist is not merely to explain the techniques and encourage members to implement them; he is to elicit discussion and comments about the techniques from the group, getting members to talk specifically about how they can use the technique.

Building Positive Associations
Concerning Eating Control

The therapist explains that the purpose of this program is neither to put participants on a diet nor to take away their eating pleasures. On the contrary, the program is designed to add to their pleasure of eating by teaching them to eat properly and to eat intentionally like a gourmet, one who really enjoys her food to the fullest with all of her senses (visual, olfactory, tactile, gustatory). One who eats indiscriminately just stuffs food hastily into her mouth without really enjoying the eating experience. By changing one's eating habits, one can "eat less but enjoy it more." One can learn to enjoy food by looking at it, appreciating the coloring of the food and its arrangement and enjoying its aroma. Most importantly, one can learn to eat slowly and enjoy each *small* mouthful with her lips and teeth. The taste and texture of the food can be more fully enjoyed by chewing the food thoroughly, using the taste buds on the right side of the tongue, the left side, and then the back of the tongue before swallowing. To fully enjoy food this way, one must eat slowly and obtain more oral gratification with less food by using more lip and chewing movements. The purpose of this program, then, is not to deprive individuals of their pleasure but to increase those pleasures. By changing eating patterns to consume fewer calories, one can at the same time learn to enjoy eating more.

Participants, then, are to EAT INTENTIONALLY. When they are eating, they should do nothing else (no studying, no reading, no watching TV). Eating is to be dissociated from other activities. When the individual eats, she should enjoy it to the fullest and let nothing distract her. By doing nothing else while eating, the participant can learn to enjoy eating more; also stimuli from other activities lose their control in initiating the chain of behaviors and conditions that terminate in eating. When one eats intentionally, she should relish every mouthful. If she is going to eat, she should enjoy it. Such a procedure brings eating behavior under the control of one's intentions, helps break associations between eating and other behaviors, and slows the rate of eating.

Individuals should not consider themselves on a diet. By dieting we frequently mean eating only certain low-calorie foods in order to lose weight. Dieting and changing eating patterns are not the same thing. Participants should consider themselves, not as dieting, but merely as changing their eating patterns so as to achieve weight reduction and to acquire eating habits that will later enable them to remain at their desired weight and still retain the pleasures that eating affords. Too many diets consist of crash programs. Although they may effect a rapid weight loss, such a rapid weight loss increases a person's disposition to eat, and this disposition usually becomes strong enough to overcome the person's temporary motive concerning the desirability of weight loss. Many diets so severely limit the kind and amount of food a person may eat that the dieter begins to feel deprived and discouraged and finds herself breaking the diet and regaining the lost weight. A good many diets advocate foods which an individual can consume only for a limited time period (e.g., liquid diets, the grapefruit diet) and teach the person nothing about better eating habits. People lose weight only to regain it when they attempt to return to a more normal eating plan. Such diets requiring specialized foods and situations are difficult to maintain; and when eating circumstances return to normal, the individual finds herself returning to old habits and puts on weight. Other diets such as the carbohydrate diet are based upon false nutritional assumptions. It has been demonstrated that the only reason people on carbohydrate diets lose weight is because, by limiting their intake of carbohydrates, they also decrease their caloric intake. Calories are still what really counts! Furthermore, adhering to the carbohydrate diet for a long period of time can be definitely detrimental to one's health. Hence, group members are to keep in mind that, if they really want to lose weight and not regain it, they must change their eating habits in a sensible way. Developing effective self-control in the area of eating requires eating a nutritionally balanced diet daily and *learning self-control under circumstances and with foods which are to be the individual's permanent eating pattern.* Accomplishing this requires changing habits concerning *when one eats, what one eats, and how much one eats.* Well-balanced diets not only ensure good health but have the extra advantage that the individual will not have a strong craving for carbohydrates, sugars, and fats because, unlike the case in dieting with specific foods, a well-balanced diet allows the person to eat an appropriate amount of these foods.

All the techniques to be used in this program are designed to help each person develop desirable habits concerning the WHEN, WHAT, and HOW MUCH of eating. Participants will learn to eat sensibly and really enjoy eating. By gradually learning to change their food habits, they won't feel deprived but rather will find themselves "Eating less, but enjoying it more." Developing self-control over the WHEN, WHAT, and HOW MUCH of eating doesn't mean that the person will *never* have a between-meal snack, or *never* have a second helping. Rather, it means that, in general, she will be able to fit such eating occasions into an all-round pattern of appropriate eating habits which promote weight control and help the subject learn really to enjoy food, not just gulp it down. The goal of the program is not simply to aid patients with weight reduction but to enable them to learn new eating patterns which will be lasting and satisfying habits. This program, then, does not prescribe a diet, and participants should not constantly talk with others about dieting, as such conversation tends to make one feel deprived of eating pleasures and misses the purpose of the present program—developing new eating habits.

Shaping Behavior

The participants are to be instructed how to use a shaping procedure to modify their eating patterns. The importance of small steps and realistic goals in developing more appropriate eating behavior should be emphasized throughout *all* sessions. Developing more self-control of eating behavior is a gradual process involving the planning of goals which are limited enough to be realistic. Behavior should be changed gradually so that the changed behavior will be reinforced. Changed eating behavior should be planned for hierarchies of situations which gradually increase in difficulty within a framework of realistic goals and self-rewards. Some methods of shaping behavior follow.

1. Set goals only for each day and each moment (e.g., no snacks this morning; no eating in my room).

2. List situations in which one eats most, and stop eating in some of these situations, first concentrating on situations in which it will be easiest not to eat.

3. Before attending social events, determine how much one will eat (e.g., only twelve peanuts and one slice of cake; only one piece of pizza).

4. Do something incompatible with eating when in a situation in which one tends to eat (e.g., file nails while watching TV).

5. Use aids to help one not to eat. Smoke a cigarette, chew gum, have a noncaloric Life Saver.

6. List the situations in which one eats less, and further decrease and finally eliminate eating in these situations (e.g., no refreshments at movies or ball games).

7. Limit between-meal eating to certain specified foods. For example, after-class snacks can be limited to diet cola or coffee with an artificial sweetener. When the girls go out to have a snack, one can order a salad or a dish of fruit. If a fountain doesn't have diet cola, one can order a coke and drink only half of it (Waste the money—that's better than acquiring fat!).

8. List the activities and situations in which one doesn't eat and then engage in those activities more often and enter those situations more frequently (e.g., study in the library where one cannot eat; if one doesn't eat while writing, start studying with a pencil in hand and write study notes).

9. Control between-meal snacking by gradually lengthening periods of abstention, working first with periods of the day that cause least difficulty in the temptation to overeat. When one has succeeded in abstaining a specified period of time, allow a highly rewarding food at the end of that time. But the amount to be eaten should be determined beforehand.

The therapist should help individual members decide how best to start shaping their own eating behavior toward the establishment of appropriate eating habits. The emphasis should be on gradualness and realistic goals.

Keeping Records of Eating Behavior

Each participant can be given a small notebook which she can carry in her purse. In the notebook she is to record every day: the food eaten, the amount, the number of calories consumed, the occasion (e.g., breakfast, study break, after-class snack), what happened before eating, what happened after eating, any particular emotional feeling at the time (e.g., tense, blue, tired), and the total amount of calories consumed each week. Recording eating behavior is to be used as both an assessment and treatment technique. As an assessment technique, the records should help identify the current discriminative, eliciting, and reinforcing stimuli associated with the eating behavior. Since from the first session the therapist will be asking participants to lose at least 2 pounds a week, participants should be instructed that for the first three weeks they should make records not only of the occurrence of eating but also of times they were tempted to eat but didn't because of their commitment to lose weight. In recording times they resisted eating, they should list: the food desired, the occasion, what happened before the temptation to eat, what they did instead of eating, what happened after resisting the temptation, and any emotional feeling experienced when tempted to eat. Records of actual eating behavior should be kept throughout the program and such records consulted at the beginning of each discussion period. The records will serve as a treatment technique since recording will aid participants in cutting down on food when they realize how much they actually eat. Such recording actually takes little time and, with moderate eating, such record-keeping becomes very simple. The heavy eater and the frequent snacker will, of course, have to record more than the controlled eater. Most participants will find that, in order to lose weight, their total daily intake will need to be reduced to between 1,000 to 1,500 calories. One pound of fat is equivalent to approximately 3,500 calories. Thus, in order to lose 2 pounds a week, an individual must reduce her weekly calorie consumption to 7,000 calories below that needed to provide energy for normal activities while keeping body weight constant. A woman who is moderately active needs about 1,800 to 2,400 calories per day to sustain normal activity and body weight. Therefore, in order to lose 2 pounds a week, most women will have to decrease their intake to about 1,000 to 1,500 calories daily. Daily intakes above 1,600 calories give such slow results in weight loss as to be too discouraging. Once a person achieves her desirable weight she can, of course, gradually increase daily caloric intake to the point where she observes that her weight remains constant.

Participants should learn an active verbal repertoire with which they can translate caloric intake into ultimate body fat. They should learn the caloric values of different kinds of foods. For example, an average piece of pie (approximately 275 calories) is equal to about one-tenth of a pound of fat. Pie has approximately the same number of calories as a baked potato with a pat of butter and a small serving of steak. Also, for example, two pieces of fudge (220 calories) are equivalent in calories to three medium-sized apples (225 calories). Such a procedure helps the participants become more calorie conscious. Keeping records of food intake helps them discriminate situations in which they tend to eat, helps them become more fully aware of their eating habits, and aids them in learning to eat on purpose.

Weight loss usually doesn't proceed evenly, and some weeks may show more loss than others although the person is decreasing her caloric consumption by the same amount. In general, though, an average weight loss of 2 pounds a week can be steadily maintained.

The records will be discussed and evaluated during discussion periods, and suggestions appropriate to more desirable habits concerning the WHEN, WHAT, and HOW MUCH of eating will be made. Discussion will also revolve around the degree of hunger when the food was eaten, how satisfying the food was, the emotional feelings before eating, how easily one could have not eaten, and how this might have been successfully accomplished.

Developing Appropriate Stimulus Control of Eating Behavior

This technique will be given formal introduction in this session, but throughout remaining sessions participants will be aided in using shaping to narrow the range of stimuli which control eating.

Certain situations present the stimuli for a person's eating behavior. One can modify her eating patterns by either changing these stimuli or by changing the behavior that occurs in certain stimulus situations. Participants should be instructed to select carefully the stimuli that are to control their eating behavior. This can be accomplished in a number of ways:

Narrowing the Range of Stimuli Which Control Eating

People with weight problems frequently eat in a large variety of circumstances. One way to control eating is to limit the situations in which eating is allowed to occur. When the participant eats, she should do that and nothing else. The subject should not allow herself to engage in other activities (e.g., studying, reading, watching TV) while eating. At home, the person should see to it that eating can occur only in certain places, as at the kitchen table, for example, or only in the dorm lounge and not in the dorm room. Temporal control over eating can be developed by specifying a time for eating meals and sticking to that time. The patient is not to skip meals but to eat them at a regular time. Following a strict temporal pattern for eating usually results in feelings of hunger disappearing except just before mealtime. Women having difficulty restricting their eating to meals should arrange a *routine* extra feeding, such as milk and crackers or vanilla wafers. These should always be taken at the same specified time, however.

The main goal in establishing appropriate stimulus control of eating is to bring eating under the control of stimuli that occur infrequently in the participant's normal activities. Hence, eating should be dissociated from the routine activities of the day. Each participant can discover the stimuli which mark the occasion for her eating and can change these stimuli. She may do this in many ways: seeing that snacks are not around; not walking home past the bakery; shopping only from a list which is prepared after a satisfying meal; not lingering at the table after a meal; going for a walk during a study break insteak of making a trip to the snack-vending machines; working, studying, and relaxing in places where eating is not allowed or is less likely to occur; not carrying money for between-meal snacks; and if a snack such as a candy bar is bought, it should be broken into small pieces and placed in an inconvenient place. The client should also gradually restrict the situations in which she allows herself to eat.

Highlighting the Stimuli Associated with Appropriate Eating

Participants are to be encouraged to allow eating to occur only in the presence of certain stimuli. Such stimuli can include a temporal pattern or a particular place or the stimuli of particular items. For example, the client can specify that she will never snack till at least three hours after meals. She may make a rule never to eat unless she is sitting at a table. Individuals can decide to limit between-meal snacks only to specified foods such as apples, vanilla wafers, celery sticks, or carrot sticks. By specifying the stimuli under which she will allow herself to eat, the individual will find that she is less tempted to eat under other circumstances; and if she does eat in response to stimuli other than the ones she has designated as appropriate, she will feel guilty.

Manipulating Deprivation and Satiation

It is important that the participant does not severely deprive herself but rather embarks upon a gradual program of weight reduction. Food intake should be planned to avoid long periods of deprivation and to help the client through difficult periods. Also keeping other needs satisfied will reduce hunger. Participants can also eat nonfattening foods (e.g., orange, apple, cracker) after brief periods of abstention.Participants can arrange to have highly desirable foods available only when hunger is low (e.g., encountering desserts only at the end of meals) and less desirable foods available when hunger is high (e.g., Rye-Krisp only for between-meal snacks). It may also be helpful to eat a bit of filling food just before entering a situation in which she will have a strong tendency to eat (e.g., 6 ounces of juice or milk just before mealtime or attendance at a party). Participants should be discouraged from losing weight too fast (e.g., more than 5 or 6 pounds per week) because a very rapid loss produces a level of deprivation and a disposition to eat which exceed the existing self-control. Also participants are to be discouraged from limiting the diet to one specified food such as protein because such a diet will likely produce a heightened disposition to eat other food. A well-balanced diet will have an adequate satiety value. Most-liked foods should be eaten when deprivation is less, and less-satisfying but filling foods eaten when deprivation is higher. During a meal the participant can practice eating least-desirable foods first and the most desirable ones last.

Rewarding Oneself for the Development of Self-Control

It is important that the participant reinforce herself for the development of self-control in the area of eating, or the developing self-control behavior will cease, especially since the reinforcing consequence of weight loss is accomplished slowly. Food itself is highly rewarding, and it is mandatory that the participant find powerful rewards for her behavior of not eating. Participants are to construct a list of ways by which they can reward themselves for not eating and to bring this list to the session for discussion. To reward herself for the development of self-control, she should set limited and realistic goals and make a reward contract with herself for accomplishing the goal (e.g., "If I have a salad for lunch, I'll allow myself to read an interesting novel for one-half hour"; "If I eliminate all evening snacking this week, I'll treat myself to a movie Friday night"; "If I keep supper to 600 calories, I'll allow myself to watch a TV program during a study break this evening"; "If I have a fruit salad for lunch, I'll allow myself a piece of pizza at the party tonight").

Another helpful procedure is to have the participant develop reinforcers that remove her from situations in which she is tempted to eat. For example, instead of stopping after class for a snack, she goes to her room and relaxes by listening to her stereo. If the participant tends to watch TV and eat on Friday nights, she can arrange to attend a movie or play, having decided beforehand that she won't buy refreshments there.

Participants should also be encouraged to set up a self-reward system for long-term maintenance of self-control. For example, she can make a chart and give herself an X for each day she has limited her caloric intake below 1,500 calories. For every ten X's she earns, she can buy a new stereo record. Or she may reward herself for every 5-pound loss by treating herself to a nice restaurant dinner (she should see to it that she has a small breakfast and lunch that day, however, so that her total caloric intake for that day is not excessive). She may also place twenty-five or fifty cents in a jar for each day that she successfully limits her caloric intake, and use this money to purchase some desired object. The therapist should encourage group discussion of how each individual might establish an effective reward system for the development of self-control of eating behavior.

Developing Personally Meaningful Ultimate Aversive Consequences of Overeating

Each participant should develop and write out a rather long list (at least ten) of the Ultimate Aversive Consequences (UAC's) of overeating and being fat. The trouble with overeating is that its undesirable consequences are far removed in time from the act of overeating. When a person is in a stimulus situation which tempts her to eat, she usually is not seriously contemplating the undesirable consequences that will later befall her because of her indiscriminate eating. However, if an individual can seriously contemplate and mentally rehearse these UAC's at the time a stimulus to eat inappropriately presents itself, these UAC's will serve to punish thoughts about overeating, and the actual behavior of overeating in such situations will be less likely to occur. Also if an individual actually has overeaten, immediate mental rehearsal and contemplation of the UAC's of this behavior will operate to make the individual feel guilty about overeating, making it less likely to happen again. It is important that the client *not* rehearse the UAC's before actual appropriate eating because such a practice may invite adaptation to the aversive properties of the UAC's.

In composing her list, each member is to list UAC's which are specific and meaningful to her rather than generalized abstract statements (e.g., "Overweight women die younger"; "Overweight girls aren't popular dates"). Verbal descriptions of aversive consequences the participants have actually experienced and are experiencing currently can be quite compelling (e.g., "Last summer some boys snickered at me when I appeared at the pool in my bathing suit"). Statements of actual or imagined social rejection, sarcastic treatment, critical references to bodily contours or proportions, extreme personal sensitivity over excess weight, demeaning inferences concerning professional incompetance or carelessness can all be effective (e.g., "When I wear shorts, my legs look like hams"; "That blind date never asked fat me out again"; "My mother-in-law's subtle sarcasm came through with 'You sure do love to eat, don't you, Betty?' "; "Because I choose to overeat, my Saturday night date is the TV set"; "My being overweight narrows my chances of getting married"; "People feel I'm sloppy because I'm overweight; "Because I'm fat, my friends kid me about being carefree and irresponsible").

Participants are to memorize a large repertory of UAC's and to mentally rehearse them in situations in which they are tempted to eat or immediately after they have eaten inappropriately. They should carry the list and rehearse the UAC's frequently but should not rehearse the UAC's prior to appropriate eating.

Members should also be encouraged to keep an unflattering snapshot of themselves or of a very fat person in their purse and to view it often throughout the day, telling themselves that this is the high price they are paying for inappropriate eating. They should contemplate this picture when they encounter a situation in which they are tempted to eat inappropriately or immediately after indiscriminate eating.

The UAC's can thus serve as a punishment technique as the individual thinks of the ridicule, deprivation of sexual and social satisfactions, etc., resulting from excess weight. By saying verbal self-criticisms to herself in a situation in which she tends to eat inappropriately, she decreases the probability of her eating in such situations. Saying these self-criticisms immediately following indiscriminate eating serves to punish such behavior and reduce its future probability.

Obtaining Reinforcers from Areas of Life Other than Eating

While behavioral treatment is aimed directly at changing behavior, therapists must remember that behavior is to be broadly defined to include not only motoric behavior but verbal and emotional behavior as well. While much attention is to be devoted to eating behavior *per se,* this does not mean that current behavior in other areas is to be ignored. Behavior therapy is to be concerned with any behavior (or lack of it) that has a relationship to the eating behavior of the participants.

One of the most important things for the therapist and patient to be aware of is that many people overeat because they are not receiving sufficient satisfaction from other areas of their life, such as studying, relationships with the opposite sex, companionship with one's own sex, recreation, leisure activities, etc. The therapist is to help each group member to survey major areas of her life, note where she is not gaining sufficient satisfaction, and help her (with the aid of the group) develop behavior that will increase her satisfactions in these areas. Participants may have to be coached in ways to make themselves more attractive to men, ways to meet men, methods for obtaining better grades, procedures for being more popular with women, methods of meeting new friends, means by which they can develop more satisfying leisure activities, means for enjoying the nonacademic aspects of college, etc. The therapist may find a number of different techniques helpful here, such as role-playing, attacking irrational ideas, assertion training, coaching, and instructing participants in a hierarchy of desirable behaviors to be learned and practiced. Helping individual participants develop and maintain reinforcements from the major aspects of their lives will comprise one of the most important tasks of the treatment. To the extent that many participants can accomplish this, they will have less need to turn to overeating as one of the major pleasures in their living pattern.

Establishing Behaviors Incompatible with Eating

The disposition to eat can be lessened by supplanting it with other activities which are incompatible with eating. The behavioral repertoire in various situations should be developed so that activities incompatible with eating become strong and the eating behavior weakened. Whenever possible, these incompatible activities should be ones that the participant finds highly reinforcing. There are many ways in which participants can implement and apply this technique:

1. Save highly reinforcing activities to be performed when there is a tendency to eat (e.g., read a favorite magazine, read a newspaper, watch a TV program, or perform other pleasant activities during study breaks).

2. When the client is tempted to eat, she can start highly reinforcing incompatible behaviors which will be aversive to interruption (e.g., going for a walk, taking a bus ride, writing a letter, washing her hair).

3. The participant can develop reinforcing incompatible behaviors to perform in group situations when others are eating. When the other girls are sitting around, chatting and eating, she can polish her nails or smoke or suck on a low-calorie Life Saver.

4. The participant can modify situations so she would "lose face" by eating in these situations. For example, she will be less likely to eat dessert if she announces to her table companions: "I've given up all desserts this week." When offered a snack at a party she can respond: "No thank you. I've eliminated between-meal snacks this week." Such statements from the participant establish situations in which it would be incompatible for her to eat.

5. The participant can have a list of other activities she can substitute for eating. In the area of recreation, she can involve herself in a card game or engage in some sport (e.g., hiking) or competi-

tive games (e.g., Ping-Pong). She can substitute work-related activities such as studying (having promised herself never to eat while studying), or ironing or doing the laundry or polishing shoes. She can choose social activities in which she will be less likely to eat, such as attending plays, movies, or concerts. She can keep her mouth busy by chewing gum or sucking dietetic hard candies or smoking. Pleasures that are incompatible with eating but appropriate and available can be substituted (e.g., sexual activity).

6. One may eat to avoid other activities which have aversive aspects. In such situations the participant should be encouraged to rehearse the UAC's of eating and to perform some other reinforcing activity.

7. The participant can enlist friends to help her lose weight. She can go over her daily caloric intake with a friend whom she's asked to approve her successes and admonish her for her failures. She can also make bets with friends that she'll lose so many pounds by a definite date.

8. It is important that the participant develop reinforcing incompatible responses which occur in response to various emotions which in the past have been followed by eating behavior. When depressed, she can phone a friend or go visiting, or force herself to watch a TV program. When angered, she should learn to assert herself appropriately rather than "brood and eat." Engaging in physical exercise can serve to combat both weight and tension (e.g., swimming).

9. The participant can respond to tension and anxiety by going through relaxation procedures (instead of eating) when she is in a situation where she can do this. After she relaxes, she can allow herself a short nap (setting the alarm to specify the length of her nap). Going through the relaxation procedure need not be confined to times when she is upset or anxious but can be used as a reinforcing break or activity to be substituted for eating, as in study breaks.

Utilizing Chaining

Chaining may be defined as a series of responses in which one response produces the stimuli for the next response. The frequency of the behavior that occurs at the end of a chain (in this case, eating) can be changed by altering the responses making up the chain. A chain can be broken or lengthened, or the consequences of certain responses in the chain can be manipulated so the end behavior of eating will occur less frequently. Some ways in which participants may utilize chaining to make eating behavior less frequent follow.

Lengthening the Chain

The participant will tend to "eat less but enjoy her food more" if she takes small bites on the fork or spoon, doesn't start chewing till the fork is put down again near the plate, and doesn't put the next biteful on the fork until the food in her mouth is chewed slowly, well, and swallowed. While doing this, she should completely relish and enjoy her food as described in the first technique under "Building Positive Associations Concerning Eating Control." The participant can learn to slow her rate of eating (and thus decrease the amount she eats) by interrupting her eating behavior with conversation or holding the food on the fork for increasingly longer periods before placing it in her mouth. These interruption procedures can first be practiced near the end of a meal, when the participant is not so hungry, and gradually be moved toward the beginning of the meal. The participant can gradually learn to eat small amounts, slowly and with great pleasure; and, to be able to stop eating at any point, she can lengthen the chain of behaviors that would terminate in inappropriate eating in many ways. The main goal is to have many steps in the sequence of actions which would have to occur between the desire to eat and the actual eating. The participant can make it inconvenient to eat inappropriately by refusing to carry money for snacks or change for vending machines. If she decides that she will do all of her snacking only at a fountain which is some distance from the dorm, she will be less likely to snack. The participant might allow only three cents per day for snacks, thus forcing herself to save several days for a coke or more days for a hamburger.

Learning to Eliminate Parts of a Chain

If the client refuses to have snacks around, she will not be able to engage in the behaviors of swallowing food. If she carries only her checkbook with her and refuses to cash a check for food, she will be less likely to eat when she goes out. By walking a route where she cannot stop for food, she will not end up eating. By going with her friends to a movie instead of to a restaurant, she also reduces the probability of her eating.

Decreasing the Reinforcement for Individual Members of a Chain

When the participant first feels the desire to eat a snack, she should go over the UAC's or look at the picture of the fat lady or at an unattractive picture of herself; she can keep a list of the UAC's in her change purse and rehearse them when she starts to get change for food. At home, the participant can paste a "fat lady" picture on the door of the refrigerator. She can make it rewarding to resist the temptation to eat. Each time she refuses a snack, she can put a quarter in one section of her purse and use this money for other pleasures (e.g., records, new clothes).

Using Supplementary Aversive Conditioning Techniques

The techniques described here are to be employed in the situation where the participant is having difficulty abstaining from eating too much highly fattening food such as nuts, candy, pastry, starches, soft drinks. These techniques can be employed to reduce the intake of those foods. She is to use these techniques only if she is eating too much of a particular fattening food and has not been able to limit eating this food by use of the other techniques. Some suggested techniques:

1. The participant should think of this food very often (fifteen to twenty times per day) and imagine *as vividly as she can* that eating this food will make her extremely nauseous. She should associate this food with images of things that make her sick to her stomach. She should tell herself that that the food will make her vomit if she eats it.

2. The participant can list the food on a card and carry it around with her. Several times each day she should take this card out (and possibly put it beside her "fat" picture) and tell herself *this* food causes her to be fat and ugly.

3. The participant can consider the taste of this tempting food

and imagine that the taste is so repulsive she cannot stand the flavor. She should vividly imagine the food tasting like something which she finds very unpleasant. She should try to convince herself that the particular food has this highly unpleasant taste. If, for example, the participant is fond of pizza, she can imagine pizza made with smelly spoiled sausage and moldy bacteria-infested crust. She should tell herself the taste of pizza is unbearable and that eating it will make her vomit. She should go through the procedure several times daily, doing it first when she is not very hungry and when the temptation to eat this favorite food is low or nonexistent, and then gradually going through this imagining exercise when she is more hungry and more tempted to eat the food.

5

The Mouthful Diet

Roy S. Fowler, Jr.

If you are reading this you are probably overweight. If you are overweight, it is unlikely that you are happy about it. You know that overeating is harmful to your health. You know that you are socially unattractive. You have probably tried one or more dieting systems and failed. You either did not lose the weight you set out to lose, or you lost the weight but did not keep it off.

The majority of people who are overweight in our society are not overweight because of lack of information. It has been my experience that most overweight people can plan a menu and calculate calories with an accuracy that rivals that of a trained dietician. This knowledge, however, does not seem to be enough. It is unfortunately characteristic of man, a so-called rational being, that information often has little or no impact upon behavior.

This Mouthful Diet system is designed for those people who eat too much, know they eat too much, but have been unable to stop overeating.

How Much Should You Eat?

The amount of food you should eat is an individual matter. This program contains no magical component which will miraculously change your individual metabolic characteristics so that you can eat as much as you wish and not gain weight. You have heard of people who can eat as much as they want and not gain weight. The important clue is the phrase "eat as much as they want."

Slim people tend not to want as much as you. Few people can eat an unlimited amount of food and still not gain. Slim people are as concerned or perhaps more concerned about their weight than is the typical obese person. It may be true that your neighbor, who is slim and attractive, is able to eat more than you and still not gain weight. There are individual differences. The important consideration at this point, however, is that you are overweight and, if you are maintaining that weight or gaining, you are probably eating too much. The fact that the amount you eat may be less than your slim neighbor eats is irrelevant. He's lucky. You're not.

Why Do You Eat?

Skinny people seem to eat for different reasons than fat people. Fat people eat in response to external cues rather than internal cues. Fat people seldom eat because they are hungry. They eat because the food looks good or because something in their environment triggers an eating response.

Skinny people seem to have an internal meter which indicates how much energy has been consumed and when it is time to put in more fuel. When enough fuel has been put in, the meter says "full," and they stop eating. Fat people either lack this internal meter or it is out of order.

Skinny people can have food around them and not eat if they are full. This is not so true of fat people. Few fat people eat large meals. Instead, they nibble little bites all the time—once they get started. Fat people are capable of eating a whole cake or two dozen cookies, but they don't do it all at once. They take a small piece or a cookie or two, eat them, and then come back for another small helping and another and another.

The Mouthful Diet system is designed to help you eat less even if your internal meter is weak or unreliable.

Who Is Fat?

Obese is a technical term which usually refers to a person who is at least 20 percent over his ideal weight, based on life insurance actuarial tables. These tables are the result of the statistical analysis of risk groups. Insurance companies have analyzed the weights of their low-risk groups and highest-risk groups, and arrived at an ideal weight range. People who weigh within the ideal weight range tend to be low-risk people and have longer life spans and fewer medical complications. Like any statistical procedure involving large groups, individual variation is great. I will not attempt to define an ideal weight for you. Consult your private physician. He can give you a goal for your weight reduction program. If you and he agree that you are overweight and that you should eat less, the Mouthful Diet should help.

Overeating Is a Habit

Overeating is a habit. Behavioral scientists have learned a great deal about habit behavior in the last twenty years. *Habits* are defined as repetitive behaviors which have become automatic. Habits are acquired through experience. We view habits as learned behaviors which follow certain systematic rules.

One rule of habit behavior is that, if the behavior is rewarded, it will tend to become stronger and, therefore, more likely to be repeated. Rewards vary from person to person. To a person who smokes, a cigarette might be a reward. To a person who does not smoke, it would not be. To the drinker, a drink is a reward.

Because rewards strengthen or reinforce the behavior which they follow, we call them "reinforcers." To most fat people, food is a powerful reinforcer. Eating makes more eating likely if food is a reward. Obviously one has to eat, so it is important to try to control the rewarding or reinforcing aspects of food.

Reinforcers have the most impact if they are immediate. Putting it another way, a reinforcer, like a carrot dangling in front of a donkey, will work best if it is on a short stick. When you eat a bite of tasty food, it immediately reinforces eating. If it tastes very good, you are quite likely to take another bite. The reinforcer for not eating, however, tends to be on a very long stick. It takes a long time, for example, to fit into that new bikini you have admired, or to get into a size smaller suit, or to look the way you looked at high school graduation. It is little wonder, then, that reminders of how great it would be to lose weight prove unable to compete with the immediate reinforcement of that delicious mouthful of food.

Deprivation and Dieting

In addition to the above characteristics of reinforcement, we have also learned what happens to reinforcers after deprivation. Deprivation means going without. Probably you all have had the experience of a period of dieting followed by a binge of overeating. This is understandable when you recognize that deprivation makes reinforcers more powerful. The longer you go without a reinforcer, the more powerful that reinforcer becomes. Food is something you cannot go without forever. After a period of deprivation, you'll eventually discover that you have to eat something. When you do eat, you will discover that food has become even more reinforcing than it was before dieting.

The reinforcement-enhancing characteristics of deprivation help explain the failures of such popular dieting techniques as the "fad food" diet, which involves the deprivation of all but specific foods, or the "crash diet," which involves deprivation of all foods.

If you deprive yourself of foods which you especially like (for example, high-calorie foods such as cookies or a hot-fudge sundae), there will probably come a time when a hot fudge sundae or a cookie is so potent a reinforcer that it will overcome any of your resolutions to swear off goodies. I feel that it is important to eat a well-balanced diet, and this should include foods which you like even if they are goodies with high caloric value. You should include goodies in your diet and learn to control them. The Mouthful Diet will help you gain control of goodies rather than have goodies control you.

I am also opposed to starvation or crash dieting. If you try starvation dieting, you will soon discover that any kind of food takes on a fantastically powerful reinforcing quality. You may find yourself, therefore, gaining weight more rapidly after a crash diet than before. This may also explain another characteristic eating pattern of fat people. They eat sparingly for breakfast, sparingly for lunch, and continuously in the evening; in other words there is deprivation in the morning, deprivation at noon, and loss of control in the evening.

You should not attempt to lose weight quickly. I regard a weight loss of between 1 and 2 pounds per week as ideal. If you lose any faster, it means that you are depriving yourself too rapidly, and food is likely to become so reinforcing that it will overwhelm your self-control. You need to learn to eat food in a controlled manner so that when you have lost the weight you desire, you will have established an eating habit pattern which you can maintain. Starving yourself is going to produce a habit pattern which can not be maintained.

The closer the eating pattern established during dieting is to a reasonable maintenance diet, the more likely you are to maintain that pattern after you reach your ideal weight.

Goals of the Mouthful Diet

The Mouthful Diet is a habit control system. If you follow the instructions, you should:

1. Lose weight gradually but steadily over a long period of time.
2. Break up and weaken the automatic aspects of your overeating.
3. Increase your self-control.
4. Learn to control the amount of food you eat.
5. Establish an eating pattern which you will be able to maintain.

This is a do-it-yourself program. You should need very little professional assistance. However, anyone who embarks upon a diet program should see his physician for periodic evaluations of his medical status.

Starting the Diet

The first step is to gather baseline or starting point information about how much you eat and how this relates to your weight. Notice that I said "how much," not "what" you eat. You are to keep a food consumption record for one week before you start any special effort at cutting down. This is easy to do and involves counting every mouthful of food as you take it. Your instructions are to:

1. *Count every mouthful of food and every swallow of caloric liquid.* The size of the bite is relatively unimportant, as is the content. You need not count water, black coffee, or tea without cream and sugar. You must count liquor, fruit juices, milk, soft drinks, and coffee or tea with cream or sugar.

2. *Count every mouthful as you take it.* This will tend to break up the automatic pattern of eating, and it will slow you down. Don't take several bites and then count in a flurry. Count after every bite. In order to count immediately, it will be necessary for you to purchase a tally counter. Several types are available. Most dieters have found that a golf counter which fits on the wrist like a wrist watch is the most convenient, and won't get lost in purses. Golf counters can be found at most sporting goods stores or pro shops. Don't try to keep a tally on a piece of paper. It is too much work, and the paper gets lost. Buy a counter even if it is a fifty-cent, plastic, grocery bill counter.

3. *Keep daily records of mouthful counts.* From your record of counts, you will derive an individual program of daily upper limits which will help you to exercise self-control while gradually reducing weight and intake. For your convenience, a baseline record-keeping form is provided (figure 5-1).

4. *Weigh yourself before you start counting, and weigh yourself one week later.* It is important that you weigh yourself at the same time of day because there are weight fluctuations throughout the day. You will probably weigh less in the morning than in the evening. Make sure that you are wearing about the same amount of clothes every time you weigh. Be sure that you use the same scales every time you weigh. It is acceptable to use bathroom scales if you first check to see that they are reliable. This doesn't mean that they have to be in exact agreement with your doctor's scales. It means that, if you weigh yourself now and then again in two or three minutes, the weight should be the same. Some scales are not reliable, and you can weigh yourself five times in an hour and get five different weights. If this happens, it is important to buy new scales. Your scales may be off several pounds in comparison with your doctor's scales. His are probably more accurate than yours; but if your scales always produce the same error, you can still accurately measure the change that takes place over a length of time.

Figure 5-1 Baseline Week Weight-Mouthful Record

WEIGHT AT THE START OF THE WEEK_____(No. 1)

DATE_____MOUTHFULS TAKEN_____

1._____(No. 2)   _____(No. 3)

2._____(No. 4)   _____(No. 5)

3._____(No. 6)   _____(No. 7)

4._____(No. 8)   _____(No. 9)

5._____(No. 10)   _____(No. 11)

6._____(No. 12)   _____(No. 13)

7._____(No. 14)   _____(No. 15)

         TOTAL MOUTHFULS FOR THE WEEK_____(No. 16)

         AVERAGE (TOTAL ÷ 7)_____(No. 17)

WEIGHT AT START OF WEEK_____(No. 18) (Same as No. 1)

WEIGHT AT END OF WEEK_____(No. 19)

DIFFERENCE IN WEIGHT_____(No. 20)

Using the Baseline Record Form

Weigh yourself and record your weight at the top of the page in box No. 1. Write the date that you start counting in box No. 2. At the end of the first day's counting, you should record in box No. 3 the total number of bites taken that day. Write the date of the second day of counting in box No. 4. Record in box No. 5 the second day's total count of mouthfuls taken. Keep this up for the rest of the week. Be sure to start each day's counting by setting your counter back to 0; then keep accumulating your total throughout the day. Repeat this procedure each day for the rest of the week. At the end of the week, your record should look something like figure 5-2.

It is now time to see what simply counting mouthfuls has done to your weight. If you have been eating in your normal fashion, you should *not* have lost weight. However, in our experience many people find that they have already started to cut down.

To measure the change, write your weight at the start of the baseline week in box No. 18. Then weigh yourself in the morning following the completion of the baseline week. Record that weight in box No. 19. Any difference between the two weights should be recorded in box No. 20. This tells you how much weight you have gained or lost during the baseline week. The completed baseline record should look like figure 5-3.

From your baseline record you learn:

1. How much weight you have lost or gained.
2. What your average total number of mouthfuls was for the week.
3. The effect of this number of mouthfuls in terms of weight change.

If you gained weight, obviously you are going to have to eat fewer bites. If you lost weight, then you are on the right track. I feel that a weight loss of between 1 and 2 pounds per week is the ideal rate. If you are losing more rapidly, you are not eating enough. Use the baseline record to calculate the upper limit you should set for yourself in the second week. To help you keep track of your upper-limits or mouthfuls allowance, use the weekly weight-mouthful record (figure 5-4).

Figure 5-2 Baseline Week Weight-Mouthful Record (Interim)

WEIGHT AT THE START OF THE WEEK __187 lbs_ (No. 1)

DATE   MOUTHFULS TAKEN

1.____May 11_____(No. 2)   ____132_____(No. 3)

2.____May 12_____(No. 4)   ____85_____(No. 5)

3.____May 13_____(No. 6)   ____115_____(No. 7)

4.____May 14_____(No. 8)   ____118_____(No. 9)

5.____May 15_____(No. 10)   ____120_____(No. 11)

6.____May 16_____(No. 12)   ____80_____(No. 13)

7.____May 17_____(No. 14)   ____120_____(No. 15)

                TOTAL MOUTHFULS FOR THE WEEK_____(No. 16)
                        AVERAGE (TOTAL ÷ 7)_____(No. 17)
        WEIGHT AT START OF WEEK_____(No. 18) (Same as No. 1)
        WEIGHT AT END OF WEEK_____(No. 19)
        DIFFERENCE IN WEIGHT_____(No. 20)

The Mouthful Diet

Figure 5-3 Baseline Week Weight-Mouthful Record (Completed)

WEIGHT AT THE START OF THE WEEK___187 lbs (No. 1)

DATE_____ MOUTHFULS TAKEN_____

1.___May 11_____(No. 2)   132_____(No. 3)

2.___May 12_____(No. 4)   85_____(No. 5)

3.___May 13_____(No. 6)   115_____(No. 7)

4.___May 14_____(No. 8)   118_____(No. 9)

5.___May 15_____(No. 10)   120_____(No. 11)

6.___May 16_____(No. 12)   80_____(No. 13)

7.___May 17_____(No. 14)   120_____(No. 15)

TOTAL MOUTHFULS FOR THE WEEK___770_____(No. 16)

AVERAGE (TOTAL ÷ 7)_____110_____(No. 17)

WEIGHT AT START OF WEEK___187___(No. 18) (Same as No. 1)

WEIGHT AT END OF WEEK___187___(No. 19)

DIFFERENCE IN WEIGHT___0___(No. 20)

Figure 5-4 Weekly Weight-Mouthful Record

WEEK____1____(No. 1)

CURRENT RECORD FOR WEEK

DATE		UPPER LIMIT MOUTHFULS		ACTUAL MOUTHFULS	
1._____	(No. 2)	_____	(No. 9)	_____	(No. 16)
2._____	(No. 3)	_____	(No. 10)	_____	(No. 17)
3._____	(No. 4)	_____	(No. 11)	_____	(No. 18)
4._____	(No. 5)	_____	(No. 12)	_____	(No. 19)
5._____	(No. 6)	_____	(No. 13)	_____	(No. 20)
6._____	(No. 7)	_____	(No. 14)	_____	(No. 21)
7._____	(No. 8)	_____	(No. 15)	_____	(No. 22)
		TOTAL		_____	(No. 23)
		AVERAGE		_____	(No. 24)

Weight at start of week_____(No. 25)

Weight at end of week _____(No. 26)

Difference between the above two weights _____(No. 27)*

*If the difference (No. 27) indicates 1 or 2 lbs. weight loss, use the average (No. 24) as your upper limit for each day next week (Nos. 9-15).

If the difference (No. 27) equals 0 or a gain in weight, subtract 2 mouthfuls each day from the average to set your upper limits (Nos. 9-15); for example: If your average was 100, you would have 100-2 = 98 for day No. 1; 98-2 = 96 for day No. 2; 96-2 = 94 for day No. 3, etc.)

If the difference (No. 27) is a loss of greater than 3 lbs. you are losing too quickly. Increase your average mouthfuls per day for the next week (no more than 2 per day).

Using the Weekly Weight-Mouthful Record

Set your upper limit according to your baseline loss or gain pattern.

You lost weight during the baseline week

If you have lost 1 or 2 pounds during your week of counting, congratulations! You cut down, and it worked. Use the average bites taken that week as your upper limit or allowance for each day this week. That is, if your average was 110 bites (as in figure 5-3) and you lost 1 or 2 pounds, you should write the number 110 as your upper limit for each day (boxes 9 through 15). Your record for this week should look like figure 5-5 before you start counting.

No weight loss

If you failed to lose or gained weight during your baseline week, then you must eat less. We have found that if you decrease your mouthful limits by 2 mouthfuls a day, you will gradually find a level at which you lose steadily. Use the average bites taken during the baseline week as your starting point and and subtract two bites a day to set your upper limits for this week. If your average was 110 bites (as in figure 5-3), your first-day limit for this week is 110-2, which is 108; second day 108-2, which is 106; third day 106-2, which is 104, etc. Your record would look like figure 5-6.

You lost too much

If the difference is a loss of more than 3 pounds, it would be a good idea to eat a little more this week. We suggest adding to your upper limit by no more than two mouthfuls a day. Your record would look like figure 5-7.

After You Have Set Your Upper Limits
for the Week

Once your limits have been set and you know if you are to eat more, less, or the same this week, you should keep counting each day and record the actual number of mouthfuls taken per day in boxes 16–

Figure 5-5   Weekly Weight-Mouthful Record
              (You lost 1–2 pounds last week)

WEEK_____1_____(No. 1)

CURRENT RECORD FOR WEEK

DATE			UPPER LIMIT MOUTHFULS			ACTUAL MOUTHFULS	
1.	May 18	(No. 2)	110	(No. 9)			(No. 16)
2.	May 19	(No. 3)	110	(No. 10)			(No. 17)
3.	May 20	(No. 4)	110	(No. 11)			(No. 18)
4.	May 21	(No. 5)	110	(No. 12)			(No. 19)
5.	May 22	(No. 6)	110	(No. 13)			(No. 20)
6.	May 23	(No. 7)	110	(No. 14)			(No. 21)
7.	May 24	(No. 8)	110	(No. 15)			(No. 22)
			TOTAL				(No. 23)
			AVERAGE				(No. 24)

Weight at start of week____185____(No. 25)

Weight at end of week _____(No. 26)

Difference between the above two weights _____(No. 27)*

*If the difference (No. 27) indicates 1 or 2 lbs. weight loss, use
the average (No. 24) as your upper limit for each day next week
(Nos. 9-15).

If the difference (No. 27) equals 0 or a gain in weight, subtract
2 mouthfuls each day for the average to set your upper limits
(Nos. 9-15); for example: If your average was 100, you would have
100-2 = 98 for day No. 1; 98-2 = 96 for day No. 2; 96-2 = 94 for
day No. 3, etc.)

If the difference (No. 27) is a loss of greater than 3 lbs. you
are losing too quickly. Increase your average mouthfuls per day
for the next week (no more than 2 per day).

Figure 5-6 Weekly Weight-Mouthful Record
(You did not lose last week)

WEEK____1____(No. 1)

CURRENT RECORD FOR WEEK

DATE		UPPER LIMIT MOUTHFULS		ACTUAL MOUTHFULS	
1.__May 18__(No. 2)		__108__(No. 9)		____(No.16)	
2.__May 19__(No. 3)		__106__(No. 10)		____(No. 17)	
3.__May 20__(No. 4)		__104__(No. 11)		____(No. 18)	
4.__May 21__(No. 5)		__102__(No. 12)		____(No. 19)	
5.__May 22__(No. 6)		__100__(No. 13)		____(No. 20)	
6.__May 23__(No. 7)		__98__(No. 14)		____(No. 21)	
7.__May 24__(No. 8)		__96__(No. 15)		____(No. 22)	
		TOTAL		____(No. 23)	
		AVERAGE		____(No. 24)	

Weight at start of week____187____(No. 25)

Weight at end of week _____(No. 26)

Difference between the above two weights _____(No. 27)*

*If the difference (No. 27) indicates 1 or 2 lbs. weight loss, use the average (No. 24) as your upper limit for each day next week (Nos. 9-15).

If the difference (No. 27) equals 0 or a gain in weight, subtract 2 mouthfuls each day for the average to set your upper limits (Nos. 9-15); for example: If your average was 100, you would have 100-2 = 98 for day No. 1; 98-2 for day No. 2; 96-2 = 94 for day No. 3, etc.)

If the difference (No. 27) is a loss of greater than 3 lbs. you are losing too quickly. Increase your average mouthfuls per day for the next week (no more than 2 per day).

Figure 5-7   Weekly Weight-Mouthful Record
               (You lost too much last week)

WEEK_____1_____(No. 1)

CURRENT RECORD FOR WEEK

DATE	UPPER LIMIT MOUTHFULS	ACTUAL MOUTHFULS
1.___May 18___(No. 2)	___112___(No. 9)	_____(No. 16)
2.___May 19___(No. 3)	___114___(No. 10)	_____(No. 17)
3.___May 20___(No. 4)	___116___(No. 11)	_____(No. 18)
4.___May 21___(No. 5)	___118___(No. 12)	_____(No. 19)
5.___May 22___(No. 6)	___120___(No. 13)	_____(No. 20)
6.___May 23___(No. 7)	___122___(No. 14)	_____(No. 21)
7.___May 24___(No. 8)	___124___(No. 15)	_____(No. 22)
	TOTAL	_____(No. 23)
	AVERAGE	_____(No. 24)

Weight at start of week____180____(No. 25)

Weight at end of week _____(No. 26)

Difference between the above two weights _____(No. 27)*

*If the difference (No. 27) indicates 1 or 2 lbs. weight loss, use
the average (No. 24) as your upper limit for each day next week
(Nos. 9-15).

If the difference (No. 27) equals 0 or a gain in weight, subtract
2 mouthfuls each day for the average to set your upper limits
(Nos. 9-15); for example: If your average was 100, you would have
100-2 = 98 for day No. 1; 98-2 for day No. 2; 96-2 = 94 for day
No. 3, etc.)

If the difference (No. 27) is a loss of greater than 3 lbs. you
are losing too quickly. Increase your average mouthfuls per day
for the next week (no more than 2 per day).

22. You may eat fewer mouthfuls than your upper limit but, of course, not more. At the end of the week, you should calculate your average mouthfuls taken this week; and, on the basis of weight change, set your upper limit for the next week.

Common Problems: I'm Counting But Not Losing Weight

I believe that it is important for you to practice self-control in small steps. The self-control muscle (figuratively speaking) is exercised every time you stop eating when you would like to continue. As with a muscle, if you try to exercise it too much before you have built up strength, you can expect it to fail or become weakened. I believe in gradual exercise and slow strengthening. At first you may find that you are following instructions and are stopping when you reach your upper limit, but in spite of that you are not yet losing weight. That is all right because during the first part of the program you are still searching for the upper-limit level which will allow you to lose weight in a consistent fashion. Some people may have to cut down the number of mouthfuls they take by as much as two-thirds of the baseline mouthfuls. If this is true, then it will take you several weeks of gradually cutting down before you find the loss level.

However, if you are following instructions and stopping at the upper limit you have set for yourself, you are still exercising the self-control muscle. *Learning to stop eating is the most difficult part of dieting.* When you have practiced stopping frequently enough, it becomes easier to continue this pattern. At first, stopping at bite 150 is as difficult, if not more difficult, than stopping at bite 75 or less later on. This is especially true when you stop and don't see weight loss. Don't give up. Keep cutting down and keep stopping. You are rehearsing the behavior which is going to make the difference later. You are controlling your own eating behavior. You are stopping when you don't want to stop.

Bite Size

You will probably find that as you become more consistent in counting mouthfuls and as the number you allow yourself goes down, the size of your mouthfuls increases. Some people have very large mouths and try to take as large a bite as possible. That's all right because sooner or later you will find that there is an absolute limit to the size of bite you can take. It is also true that sooner or later you will find that taking very large bites is not very comfortable and is also unattractive. In my experience, after the first few weeks of big bites, people stop taking such large bites and go back to a more comfortable and natural pattern. It should be obvious that a few big bites equal a larger number of smaller bites if the food is the same. The amount of food and the content of food placed in the mouth make you fat. Try to find a normal eating pattern, and then adjust the amount of food you eat.

What About Special Diet Restrictions?

The mouthful diet does not tell what you can eat or what you shouldn't eat. It is assumed that you know what is good for you and what isn't. If you have any questions about what to eat, you should see a physician. If you have already seen a physician and he has placed you on a restricted diet, it doesn't necessarily mean that you cannot use the mouthful system. For example, you may be limited to a no-salt diet. All you have to do is count the food you eat and avoid food with salt. The mouthful system helps you stop eating and tells you when you have had enough. You and your physician can decide what food you should or shouldn't eat. You can then use the counting system to adjust the amount of food you eat in order to control your weight.

What To Do When Your Bites-Mouthful Allowance Gets Too Low

There is no good way to set a lower limit on the amount you should eat. If you find that your bite allowance is so low that you don't feel you are eating enough, you should look at two things:

What Are You Eating?

If you are eating mouthfuls of high caloric food, then you will need to cut down more to lose weight than your friend who takes bites of low caloric food. You may find that you are taking 50 bites a day and you not losing weight while your salad-loving neighbor is eating 200 bites and losing steadily. If you squander your mouthful allowance on goodies, you have to take fewer bites. It is, therefore, wise to eat a well-balanced diet. If you decide to switch to low-calorie food, don't cheat in advance by raising your allowance. Remember that if you lose more than 2 pounds in a week, that is the only signal to start adding to your upper limit. Don't increase your allowance before the economy dictates a change.

When Are You Eating?

The same number of mouthfuls eaten over a short period are more fattening than if they are eaten over a longer period. For example, if your upper limit is 100 mouthfuls and you eat all 100 in a few evening hours, you are less likely to lose weight than if you had eaten those 100 mouthfuls during several meals spread throughout the day. Said another way, three meals a day are better than one if the total amount of food eaten remains the same.

Specific questions about food and whether you are eating enough to avoid medical complications should be directed to your physician. *Consult your physician when you consider dieting and frequently as you diet.*

part III

supplemental
behavioral
techniques

The readings in this section describe behavioral techniques which could serve as useful adjuncts to the programs presented earlier. As a result of their comparatively limited scope, they would not be appropriate as the sole treatment method in most situations. In making use of these techniques, the therapist should consider the specific needs of the individuals to be treated as well as the relevant research pertaining to that technique. It will be apparent from a review of the material presented in chapter 2 that many questions about the applicability and effectiveness of these techniques remain to be answered.

In chapter 6 Cautela presents the rationale and procedures for covert conditioning as applied to weight control. The two primary components of this approach are covert sensitization and covert reinforcement. The reader lacking prior exposure to behavior therapy may be skeptical about the effects of imagined scenes upon actual overt behaviors. Although this is a valid concern, it should be noted that systematic desensitization, perhaps the most effective behavior therapy technique, also makes use of imagined scenes.

Experimental studies of covert sensitization as a weight control technique yield conflicting results (see chapter 2). Covert reinforcement has been the subject of fewer studies and, therefore, must be considered an interesting but unproven technique.

John and Sandra Lutzker describe a contingency contracting procedure in chapter 7. The specific directions they provide are intended for use by two people living together, one of whom desires to lose weight. It would not be difficult to modify the procedure so that a contract could be drawn up between the patient and therapist or any other cooperative person.

An implicit assumption of this type of procedure is that the patient already possesses the necessary skills for weight loss and, therefore, it is not necessary to present self-control or dietary information. In many instances this will be true; the contingency contract serves to motivate the patient to what he or she already knows how to do. If, however, the patient lacks weight control skills, contingency contracting may result in drastic measures which result in temporary weight loss rather than permanent habit change (Mann 1972).

In the context of a self-control program, contingency contracting may be useful for the patient who understands the procedures described and appears to be enthusiastic but does not seem to be able to implement the procedures with any degree of consistency. A well-designed contingency contract should help patients follow through on their commitment.

Finally, chapter 8 presents materials for an exercise management program. Mahoney (1975a) has noted that some obese individuals consume fewer calories than their normal-weight peers. Their excessive fat tissue results from extreme inactivity. In practice, the occasional obese patients who actually consume as few as 900 calories per day should not attempt to further restrict their diet. Thus the behavioral programs previously described would be inappropriate because of their focus on decreasing caloric consumption. Instead, the therapist should concentrate on increasing the energy expenditure of the patient.

In most instances, it is likely that obesity results from both overeating and underexercising. It would seem reasonable, therefore, to include exercise management routinely in behavioral weight control programs. Unfortunately, this is not usually done. With the materials presented in chapter 8, the therapist should be able to incorporate an exercise management component into the treatment program.

⑥

The Treatment
of Overeating
by Covert Conditioning

Joseph R. Cautela

A major assumption of behavior theory is that behavior is influenced by the consequences that follow the behavior. Evidence (Skinner 1969) indicates that if the frequency of a particular behavior is to be decreased, a combination of punishment for the behavior and reinforcement for antagonstic behavior is most effective.

The purpose of this chapter is to present a treatment procedure for the modification of eating behavior which punishes particular eating responses and reinforces responses antagonistic to eating. A number of studies (Ferster, Nurnberger, and Levitt 1962; Meyer and Crisp 1964; Harmatz and Lapuc 1968; Moore and Crum 1969; Upper and Newton 1971) indicate that the manipulation of the consequences of eating can be successfully employed to reduce overeating.

In the procedure to be described, both the punishing stimulus and reinforcing stimulus are presented in imagination via instructions. The method of presenting a punishing stimulus in imagina-

This chapter is reprinted with minor modifications from *Psychotherapy: Theory, Research and Practice*, 1972, *9*, 211–16. Copyright 1972 by the Division of Psychotherapy, American Psychological Association. Used with permission.

tion to decrease behavior is labeled covert sensitization (Cautela 1966, 1967). The presentation of a reinforcing stimulus in imagination is designated covert reinforcement (Cautela 1970). A major assumption of this chapter is that an aversive stimulus and a reinforcing stimulus presented in imagination via instructions have a functional relationship to covert and overt behavior as externally presented aversive and reinforcing stimuli. The assumption that covert events obey the same laws as overt events has been held by learning theorists such as Pavlov (1955, p. 285), Skinner (1969, p. 242), Kimble (1961), and Franks (1967). There is ample experimental evidence that both covert sensitization (Ashem and Donner 1968; Barlow, Leitenberg, and Agras 1969; Stuart 1967; Viernstein 1968; Wagner and Bragg, in press) and covert reinforcement (Cautela, Steffan, and Wish, in press; Cautela, Walsh, and Wish 1971; Flannery, in press; Krop, Calhoon, and Verrier 1971) are effective in the modification of behavior.

Description of Procedure

After the usual assessment procedure (Cautela 1968), the patient is given a weight questionnaire which is used to determine weight history and eating habits. The patient is also asked to write down everything he eats, including the time, place, and exact amount. He is also asked to indicate the amount of calories and grams of carbohydrates for each food item. Sometimes just recording eating behavior results in a loss of weight; but in my experience the loss is only temporary, and the patient will usually gain weight unless covert sensitization is used.

Data are accumulated for two weeks. Meanwhile during the two sessions (the patient is usually seen once a week), the patient is tested for clarity of imagery, and the Fear Survey Schedule (Wolpe and Lang 1964) and the Reinforcement Survey Schedule (Cautela and Kastenbaum 1967) are administered to determine possible aversive and reinforcing situations that may be presented in imagination.

The patient is told that overeating is a habit which gives him pleasure. The habit consists of eating too much food and food containing more fuel than is necessary to maintain his normal activity. He is told that one way to reduce his food intake is to have him associate particular eating behaviors with something unpleasant and to reward him for not engaging in the maladaptive eating behavior. He is also told that this will be done by asking him to imagine certain unpleasant and pleasant scenes. The patient is reassured that he will not develop a dislike for food in general but only for overeating and eating particular kinds of foods. The patient and therapist then agree on the desired loss of weight and keep charts on the progress of weight loss.

After the patient turns in his eating habit data on the second week, the therapist circles with a pencil the eating behavior that has to be eliminated. This behavior includes:

1. Eating between meals.
2. Eating foods with high caloric content.
3. Eating too much food at one sitting (e.g., eating two four-ounce steaks or five lamb chops or too much bread).

The patient is simply told that he is to stop engaging in these behaviors and to continue to accumulate the eating data. The patient is also asked to weigh himself every day.

At the beginning of the fourth session, the therapist indicates to the patient where he has failed to eliminate the undesirable behavior. At this time, covert sensitization and covert reinforcement are applied to those situations in which he did not eliminate the maladaptive eating behavior.

The Application of Covert Sensitization

The following instructions concern the general applications of covert sensitization given to the client:

> I am going to ask you to imagine this scene as vividly as you can. I do not want you to imagine that you are seeing yourself in these situations. I want you to imagine that you are actually in these situations. Do not only try to visualize the scenes, but try to feel, for example, the forkful of food in your hand, or the chair on which you are sitting. Actually smell the warm apple pie on the plate before you. Try to use all of your senses. The scenes I will pick are concerned with situations in which you are about to eat. It is very important that you try to visualize the scenes as clearly as possible and try to actually feel yourself in the situation.

If the client has eaten between meals, he is presented with a scene similar to the following:

> I want you to imagine that you are walking along the street and, as you pass a candy counter, you stop and pick up a few candy bars. As you begin to open the wrapper of the first bar, you get a very queasy feeling in the pit of your stomach. You start to feel weak, nauseous, and sick all over. As you raise the candy bar to your mouth, you feel a bitter liquid come up into your throat. You try to swallow it and put the candy in your mouth. As soon as the candy reaches your lips, you vomit. The vomit rushes out all over your hands, the candy, and down the front of your clothing. The sidewalk is a mess, and people stop to stare at you. Your eyes are burning, and slimy mucous continues to run down your chin and your neck. The sight of all the vomit makes you vomit even more until you cannot vomit more than a little trickle of watery substance. You feel so horrible, so sick, and so embarrassed. You turn, run away from all that mess, and feel much better.

A typical covert sensitization scene for eating highly caloric foods is as follows:

> I want you to imagine that you are at your dinner table and have just finished your first serving of steak. You reach across the table to get another piece and, just as your hand reaches the plate, you feel a queasy, churning feeling in your stomach. You transfer the steak to your plate and, just as you do, a bitter spit comes up into your throat and mouth. You swallow it and raise a piece of meat on your fork. Just as the fork reaches your lips you vomit all over your hand, all over the plate in front of you. The vomit goes all over the table and splashes on the people eating with you. They look at you horrified. You feel miserable, slimy, and the sight of the vomit mixed with food particles spread all over the table makes you vomit more and more. You hurry from the table and rush out of the room, and you feel better.

After presentation of each scene which applies to the patient, he is questioned concerning the clarity of the scene and how much discomfort he felt. If the patient reports that the scene was not clear or he could not get any discomfort from the scene, the scene is presented again in more detail. After the patient reports that the scene is clear, he is asked to carefully imagine the scene by himself. Again he is questioned concerning the clarity and degree of discomfort. He is asked to keep practicing the scene until it is clear and discomfort is experienced.

In each session, scenes are presented in which the subject gives in to the temptation to eat and vomits. Then the patient presents the same scenes to himself.

Besides the above scenes in which the client gives in to temptation, ten escape (or self-control) scenes are presented in which the client is tempted to eat, feels nauseous, and then decides not to eat. A typical escape scene:

> I want you to imagine that you have just finished eating your meal. You decide to have some dessert. As soon as you make that decision, you start to get a funny feeling in the pit of your stomach. You say, "Oh, no. I will not eat dessert." Then you immediately feel calm and comfortable.

As in the other scenes, the patient is asked to repeat the scene to himself. At the end of the session, the patient is told to practice each scene performed in the office at least twice a day at his home. He is cautioned to make the scenes as clear as possible and to include a self-control scene with each failure scene.

The patient is also instructed to say "Stop!" to himself and to imagine he is vomiting on food whenever he is tempted to eat maladaptively in real-life situations.

At each subsequent session, the patient is weighed and asked if he did all his homework. The therapist then goes over all the eating data from the previous week, and covert sensitization is applied where necessary. At this time, daily calorie and carbohydrate maximums are determined, and the patient is told not to exceed the limit set.

The Application of Covert Reinforcement

Covert reinforcement is employed to increase the probability of behaviors antagonistic to overeating.

Reinforcers are chosen from the Reinforcement Survey Schedule and from questioning the patient. The items are then tested for their reinforcing properties. The patient is asked to close his eyes and imagine that he is receiving the stimulus; e.g., if the item selected is rock and roll music, the patient is instructed in the following manner:

Choose your favorite rock and roll song—one that you know quite well—and try to imagine you really hear it. As soon as you feel that you can really hear it, signal by raising your right index finger.

The patient is then questioned about the clarity of the image. Practice receiving the reinforcer is continued until he can imagine it clearly and without any delay.

After a number of reinforcers have been chosen and tested by the patient, explain to him that these certain items or activities that give him pleasure will be paired in imagination with the behaviors that he finds difficult to do (e.g., walking away from the table after a meal). He is then instructed as follows:

In a minute I am going to ask you to try to relax and close your eyes. Then I will describe a scene to you. When you can imagine the scene as clearly as possible, raise your right index finger. I will then say the word *reinforcement.* As soon as I say the word *reinforcement,* try to imagine the reinforcing scene we practiced before—the one about your swimming on a hot day, the feeling of the refreshing water, and feeling wonderful. As soon as the reinforcing scene is clear, raise your right index finger. Do you understand the instructions? Remember to try to imagine everything as vividly as possible, as if you were really there. Now close your eyes and try to relax.

After the patient has closed his eyes and appears comfortable, the therapist presents a scene such as this one:

You are sitting at home watching TV. You say to yourself, "I think I'll have a piece of pie." You get up to go to the pantry. Then you say, "This is stupid. I don't want to be a fat pig." (Reinforcement)

Other examples of covert reinforcement scenes follow:

You are at home eating steak. You are just about to reach for your second piece, and you stop and say to yourself, "Who needs it, anyway?" (Reinforcement)

I want you to imagine that, as you eat a dish of your favorite ice cream, you see it turn to fat on your arm. (Reinforcement)

Imagine that you have lost 50 pounds and you are standing naked in front of a mirror. You congratulate yourself for getting rid of all of the flab. (Reinforcement)

As with the covert sensitization procedure, the patient is asked to practice each scene twice a day at home. Sometimes covert reinforcement is combined with covert sensitization in the following ways:

1. After the patient has imagined himself vomiting, he tells himself that doing that (i.e., giving in to temptation) was stupid and that he will not do it again, and administers a reinforcement to himself.

2. The patient imagines he is tempted to eat and feels a little nauseous but decides not to eat and feels better and administers a reinforcement to himself.

Other Procedures Combined with Covert Sensitization and Covert Reinforcement

Relaxation

If anxiety appears to be an antecedent condition to eating, the patient is taught to relax using a modified Jacobson (1938) procedure. He is taught to use relaxation as a self-control procedure (Cautela 1969). He is taught to relax before he enters into what he feels will be an anxiety-provoking situation and after he has just experienced anxiety which may still persist in part. He is also instructed to relax and covertly reinforce himself for not eating if he feels anxious and is about to eat.

Desensitization

If it is clear that specific anxiety-provoking situations are antecedent to maladaptive eating, the patient is desensitized (Wolpe 1958) to the situation. Covert reinforcement can also be used to reduce anxiety in specific situations by reinforcing antagonistic responses.

Stimulus Control

The patient is instructed to try to eat only in proper eating situations, such as in the kitchen or dining room. He is told not to eat in such situations as while watching TV or while reading, since these situations may act as stimuli for eating. In Hullian terms, they may pick up secondary-drive properties (Hull 1952); or, in operant terms, they may become discriminative stimuli for eating.

Covert Conditioning as a Self-Control Procedure

It is clear from the description of the homework assignments that the patient learns to make responses that are antagonistic to eating. Also, before the patient is discharged, he is given a weight range (e.g., 160–165 pounds). The patient is instructed to weigh himself once a week and to apply the covert conditioning procedure whenever the maximum weight is reached. The procedure is again carefully explained for possible future use.

Length of Treatment

The length of treatment, of course, depends on the desired amount of weight loss. The patient is usually seen once per week for a period of three months and then once every two weeks until the desired weight is reached. The average goal for weekly pound loss is 2 or 3 pounds.

Results

Though I have found the procedure outlined above quite effective, anecdotal results such as these are not sufficient evidence for the acceptance of the treatment procedure. The procedure is confounded by a number of interacting variables such as the behavior of the therapist, which is not specified in the procedure. Also, a combination of procedures has been used. Questions arise, such as would desensitization or covert sensitization alone be sufficient to modify maladaptive eating behavior? Of course, the questions can be properly answered by experimental analysis. Although no experimentation investigating the efficacy of combining covert sensitization and covert reinforcement to the modification of eating behavior has been completed, I am of the opinion that the procedures outlined deserve serious consideration for further investigation for the following reasons:

1. Experimental studies indicate that covert sensitization is effective in modifying other approach behaviors such as alcoholism (Ashem and Donner 1968), sexual deviation (Barlow, Leitenberg, and Agras 1969), and smoking (Wagner and Bragg, in press).

2. Studies employing covert reinforcement (Cautela, Steffan, and Wish, in press; Cautela, Walsh, and Wish 1971; Flannery, in

press; Krop, Calhoon, and Verrier 1971) indicate that it is a powerful procedure for the modification of behavior.

3. In one study (Sachs, Bean, and Morrow 1970) in which covert sensitization was compared to an operant self-control procedure in eliminating smoking behavior, covert sensitization appeared more effective.

The few studies investigating the efficacy of covert sensitization in the treatment of weight control generally report positive results. Stuart (1967) presented additional anecdotal evidence of the successful combination of covert sensitization with other operant self-control procedures in the elimination of overeating.

Ashem, Poser, and Trudall (1970) compared covert sensitization with an overt aversive stimulus in the treatment of overeating. They concluded:

> Results using covert sensitization with obesity appear good. There seems to be no need to use overt stimuli as adjuncts. Undoubtedly, results could be enhanced by conditioning a response incompatible with the compulsive eating response, once the covert sensitization has taken effect.

Sachs and Ingram (1972) found covert sensitization effective in reducing intake of selective foods.

An important question that needs experimental testing is whether the combination of covert sensitization and covert reinforcement is superfluous because maybe either of the procedures alone would be sufficient to eliminate a certain behavior. In my experience, the combination of both covert sensitization and covert reinforcement seems to hasten treatment and decrease the probability of relapse.

Problems Encountered in the Use of Covert Conditioning

A number of factors have been found to hinder the successful application of covert conditioning. These factors do not preclude the use of covert conditioning, since modification in procedure can usually eliminate or reduce the detrimental effects.

Poor Imagery

The inability to obtain clear imagery is reported by a few (about 5 percent) of the patients. They claim they cannot get sufficiently clear imagery whenever a scene is described. Usually poor imagery can be overcome by describing scenes in more detail, emphasizing the sense modality that enables the patient to get the clearest imagery, and having the client observe certain real-life situations and then try to imagine them immediately.

Ineffective Aversive Stimuli

Rarely a patient will claim that, even after very vivid and detailed description of the vomiting scenes, he never can feel nauseous or get any discomfort. For such patients, other possible aversive stimuli are chosen from the Fear Survey Schedule or from the interview situation. One patient was asked to imagine that the food was covered with worms just as she was about to eat. Another patient was asked to imagine that the food turned to blubber as it entered her body.

Incomplete Homework

Some patients report that they forget or are too busy to do the homework. It is again emphasized that homework will make treatment more effective, thereby saving them time or money. Covert reinforcement is applied by having them imagine they are practicing the procedures at home and then presenting a reinforcement.

Health Problems

Contrary to what some colleagues have expected would occur, the patients treated by covert conditioning do not lose their taste for all food. They only lose the "urge" to eat in a maladaptive manner. I also insist that every patient have a thorough physical examination before treatment is begun. This rarely has to be done, however, since by the time the clients come to me for treatment, they have made many attempts to lose weight and have had physical examinations in the process.

Summary

In summary, the covert conditioning procedure combines punishment in imagination for eating and reinforcement in imagination for responses antagonistic to eating. Often it is necessary to eliminate the drive component (anxiety) of the eating behavior. In such cases, procedures such as desensitization and relaxation are also employed.

Thus far, there have been no reported adverse effects such as *anorexia nervosa* or physical complaints. The data supporting the general effectiveness of covert sensitization and covert reinforcement as applied to other maladaptive behaviors, my experience with the techniques, and all the reports of colleagues warrant serious consideration of the procedures described in this chapter. However, hardcore experimental investigations are still needed.

7

A Two-Dimensional Contract: Weight Loss and Household Responsibility Performance

*John R. Lutzker
and Sandra Z. Lutzker*

Contingency contracting, that is, an agreement between two people to prearrange response consequences and articulate (in writing) the conditions under which the consequences will occur, has been shown to be a critical tool in behavior change strategies. Our description (1974) of how contingency contracting can be used to produce durable weight loss and an increase in household chore performance follows.

Household Contract

Any two people who share some household responsibilities can use the two-dimensional contract. Obviously, the most common pairing is husband and wife, but there are other combinations such as mother-daughter (often a nonmarried mother), roommate-roommate, father-son. If a child is a participant, he should be old enough to be entrusted with some major household responsibilities that on completion, the parent would find useful and rewarding.

This chapter is based on the authors' unpublished manuscript, 1975.

Only One Partner Needs to Desire to Lose Weight

A list of household responsibilities should be prepared by the pair. Typically, there are daily and weekly chores that need to be accomplished (see figure 7-1 for examples). Partners should be as

Figure 7-1   Assignment of Chores

Daily	Sally	Jack
Make the beds by 9:00 A.M.	Monday-Friday	Saturday-Sunday
Clean breakfast dishes	Sunday-Thursday	Friday-Saturday
Set dinner table	Tuesday, Thursday	Sunday, Monday, Wednesday, Friday, Saturday
Clear dinner table	Tuesday	Wednesday-Monday
Take out garbage	Tuesday, Thursday, Saturday	Sunday, Monday, Wednesday, Friday
Clean dinner dishes	Wednesday-Sunday	Monday, Tuesday
Sweep kitchen	Tuesday	Wednesday-Monday
Empty dishwasher	Monday-Wednesday	Thursday-Sunday
Take out newspapers		Monday-Sunday

Weekly		
Empty wastebaskets	twice weekly	twice weekly
Clean toilets	twice weekly	
Clean bathrooms	once weekly	
Clean den	once weekly	
Pick up child's room	twice weekly	
Clean kitchen floors	once weekly	
Clean sinks		once weekly
Clean mirrors		once weekly
Dust and vacuum living room		once weekly
Vacuum child's room		once weekly
Dust and vacuum master bedroom		once weekly

signed chores according to their skills, wishes, or the executed agreement. If the wife wants to lose weight, it is useful for the husband to agree to take on a few more domestic chores so that the successful completion of the household responsibility contract becomes especially rewarding to the wife. (The role of the household contract in weight loss will be covered shortly.) The chores can be distributed in any way the partners feel will ensure successful completion. For example, they might decide to have one partner do dinner dishes Monday through Friday and the other partner do them on the weekends; another arrangement could be to have one partner do the dishes on Monday, Wednesday, and Friday with the other partner doing them Tuesday, Thursday, and weekends. The object is to plan the chores with a likelihood that they will be done.

Getting the Chores Done—The Contingency

In order to keep the partners doing their chores, two steps are necessary: 1. Charts should be posted in a conspicuous place in the house and kept up to date regularly (see figures 7-2 and 7-3) regarding the completion of tasks. An X is placed on the chart when the task is completed, a minus sign is placed on the chart when the task has not been completed, and a zero is placed on the chart if doing the task was not possible, e.g., the partners went out to dinner. It is essential that the charts be kept up to date on a daily basis. 2. The number of total daily chores for each week should be counted. The sample chart in figure 7-2 for Jack shows he has 40 daily chores. Calculate 10 percent of the daily chores for one week in order to determine the number of allowable minuses for the week. That is, if there are 40 chores for the week, Jack would be allowed 4 minuses. If the person stays within his allowable number of minuses, he receives no penalty. That is, the person can simply say, "I am allowed 4 minuses and I only have 2 so far this week, so I am not going to sweep the kitchen tonight." *However,* the contingency is that, for every time that the person goes over his allotment, he must do an equal number of his partner's daily chores the following week. For example, Jack might be allowed 4 minuses (see figure 7-2). If he has 6 minuses at the end of the week (2 over his allotment), he must do 2 of Sally's daily chores the following week. If he has 10 minuses, he would have to do 6 of Sally's chores the following week. If both partners go over their minus allotment, they should still be required the next week to complete the number of their partner's chores equal to the number they went over their allotment. This contingency is an effective way of keeping the partners doing 90 percent of their agreed household chores. Most people report considerable satisfaction from this part of the contract alone. If personal schedules change or some specific chores are never getting done, then the partners should renegotiate the work contract.

Weight Contingencies

For maximum efficiency with the two-dimensional contract, it is suggested that only one partner try to lose weight at a time. (As can be seen below, if both partners gain weight while both are trying to lose at the same time, a penalty would be difficult to arrange.) Each week, on the same day, the partner who wants to lose weight must weigh-in in front of his partner. The weigh-in should be on the same scale, at the same time, in the same manner (i.e., wearing the same amount of clothes, having had or not having had a meal, etc.) every week. The weight should be recorded on a chart after each weigh-in. It is also most desirable to purchase a scale that measures weight to the nearest quarter-pound. A medical-type balance scale is preferable.

The next step for the partner who wants to lose weight is to choose a weekly criterion loss. The weekly criterion should be medically safe, and realistic. A more obese person might choose 2–3 pounds as his initial weekly criterion while a less obese person should choose ½–2 pounds as his criterion. An overall weight loss goal should also be set. Since it is usually more difficult to lose weight as the person approaches the goal, it is advisable to agree in advance that the weekly criterion be reduced after much of the weight has been lost. For example, if the wife wants to lose 30 pounds, the suggested plan would have her weekly criterion be 2 pounds per week for the first 20 pounds, 1 pound per week for the next 5 pounds, and ½ pound per week for the final 5 pounds. On the other hand, a person who only wants to lose 15 pounds should probably start with a 1-pound weekly criterion and switch to a ½-pound criterion after, perhaps, the first 8 pounds lost.

WEIGHT LOSS CONTINGENCY. Once the household contract is in effect, the partners can begin the weight program. The first weigh-in with the first weekly criterion loss should occur at the end of the first week after the household contract is in effect. The partner who is on the weight program chooses a reward to work for during that week. Figure 7-4 lists some possible rewards. It is advisable to have the person prepare his own list of potential rewards in the program. Figure 7-4, however, lists numerous rewards that have been tried by many people.

The reward should be something for which the person will work hard on weight lo ; in order to earn. As can be seen in figure 7-4, the reward can be something material such as a new piece of clothing or a record, or something nonmaterial such as a backrub or a special favor from the partner.

Figure 7-2 Jack's Chores

Daily	Mon	Tues	Wed	Thurs	Fri	Sat	Sun
Breakfast dishes					-	X	
Bed	X	X	X	-	X		
Set table	0		0		X	0	0
Clear table	0		0	X	X	0	0
Garbage	X		0		X		X
Dinner dishes	0	X					
Sweep kitchen			0	0	X	0	0
Empty dishwasher				0	0	0	X
Take out newspapers	X	X	X	-	X	X	-

Weekly							
Empty wastebaskets (twice)	X						X
Sinks (once)							X
Mirrors (once)					X		
Living room (once)					X		
Vacuum child's room (once)					X		
Bedroom (once)							X

Daily allowed minuses = 4
Weekly allowed minuses = 1

The partners should then write a brief contract stating that the person trying to lose weight will receive the reward as soon as possible after the weekly weigh-in, contingent upon reaching or falling below the prearranged weekly criterion (see figure 7-5). That is, if the person loses to the criterion or below, the reward is his. If the person does not lose to the criterion, *the reward is not forthcoming and a different reward must be chosen for the following week.* A reward that was not earned cannot be chosen again until the person has earned a different one. That is, there must be a criterion weight loss at least once before a previously ineffective reward can be tried again. How-

Figure 7-3   Sally's Chores

Daily	*Mon*	*Tues*	*Wed*	*Thurs*	*Fri*	*Sat*	*Sun*
Breakfast dishes	X	X	X	X			X
Bed						X	X
Set table		X		X			
Clear table		X	X				
Garbage		X		X	X		
Dinner dishes			X	X	X	X	X
Sweep kitchen		X					
Empty dishwasher	X	X	X				
Laundry	X	X	-	-	-	X	X

Weekly							
Empty wastebasket (twice)					X		
Toilets (twice)					X		
Bathroom (once)					X		
Refrigerator (once)							-
Den (once)						X	
Pick up child's room (twice)					X		
Kitchen (once)						X	

Daily allowed minuses = 3
Weekly allowed minuses = 2

Figure 7-4   Some Possible Rewards

Going shopping
Going to a movie, play, or concert
Going to the beach
Spending time at a favorite hobby or sport
Listening to the radio or a record
Getting to "be the boss" with partner
Spending extra time with a friend
Reading pornography
Reading or buying a desired book
Going to parties
Being alone
Goofing off
Watching TV or not watching TV
Taking a long, leisurely bubble bath
Going to class with partner
Getting a backrub from partner
Going out on the town
Making a special purchase (clothes, tools, appliance, painting, musical
    instrument, etc.)
Taking lessons in music, dance, scuba diving, etc.
Going on a picnic
Variety in sex
Sitting around reading the Sunday paper
Bouquet of fresh flowers
Going to a museum
Night out with girls/boys
Going on a trip
Going camping
Getting to sleep late
Obtaining or caring for pet(s)
Special task or favor by partner
Partner preparing a favorite dish or meal

This list was adapted in part from suggestions in Watson and Tharp (1972).

ever, successful rewards may be repeated as often as desired. Furthermore, the criterion loss is always set below the lowest previous weight. Thus, if Sally gains 5 pounds, going to 130 from her earlier low weight of 125, her next criterion for reward will be 124 pounds.

There are two critical considerations in choosing the reward. The first is that the reward be something the person really would like to have; the second is that it be something that the person can do without if it is not earned or until it is earned at a later time. Thus, sex, smoking, friendship, etc., would be poor choices because, if weight is not lost to the criterion and the reward is withheld, cheating (breaking part of the contract) will likely occur. Also, in the case of sex or friendship, the person who is not the active participant in the weight contract is penalized by his partner's failure to lose weight.

WEIGHT GAIN CONTINGENCY.   A gain is counted any time the partner weighs-in at one-quarter of a pound or more *above the previous lowest weight*. When a gain is recorded, the person does not earn the reward, and the partner *resigns* from the work contract for the full following week. That is, the person who gained weight is either left with extra chores or many of the household jobs that have been getting done will remain undone. It is important that the partner be firm in his resignation so that the resignation does act to punish weight gain.

MAINTENANCE.   Not losing but not gaining—i.e., maintenance—is neither penalized nor rewarded. Maintaining weight is certainly more desirable than gaining; however, maintaining without losing over a few weeks is not particularly desirable, so a further

Figure 7-5 Two-Dimensional Contract

Sally	Jack
will weigh-in weekly,	will be present at weekly weigh-ins,
will record data on chore charts,	will record data on chore charts,
will obtain her reward as soon as possible when earned,	will resign from this contract when appropriate,
will renegotiate this contract when necessary.	will renegotiate this contract when necessary.
signed _____	signed _____

contingency is necessary. That is, if there is no criterion weight loss for three weeks—and no gain; thus, maintenance—the penalty, the resignation contingency, is put into effect. For example, if Sally weighed 125 pounds for three straight weeks (and her criterion was 124 pounds, her husband would resign from the work contract until she lost weight to the new criterion. When she lost to 124 pounds, she would receive her reward.

Results

The first use of the two-dimensional contract was made by us in a formal research study. The wife was about 15 pounds overweight and had often lost several pounds but had never been able to maintain the loss. The contract has been in effect over two years now with desirable weight loss maintained. In addition, our household chores have been accomplished to our satisfaction as they never were prior to the contract. In fact, our formal data show that the husband did his chores only about 20 percent of the time and the wife about 60 percent of the time prior to the introduction of the household contract. Furthermore, when the chores are clearly delineated, there is no bickering about whether or not they get done or who is responsible for them since the contract covers both of those issues.

We have subsequently studied a number of other partners who used this two-dimensional contract. Most have had similar durable success and have anecdotally reported the contract has added a constructive dimension to their relationships.

Summary of Steps Necessary for a Successful Project:
    1. Delineate household chores.
    2. Make a chart for household chores.
    3. Determine the minus allotment.
    4. Determine current weight.
    5. Determine an overall weight loss goal.
    6. Determine weekly weight loss criteria.
    7. Establish weekly rewards.
    8. Implement weight contingencies.

8

Exercise Management

Genevieve Ginsburg and Jean Baker

Keeping an exercise record is simple. The purpose of this recording is to establish a baseline from which you may design a program of change for the future. Just as the input of calories can be measured when consumed in the form of food, the output can be calculated when the body is expending calories during physical activity.

A calorie is the heat needed to raise the temperature of one kilogram of water from 15 degrees to 16 degrees centigrade. In figuring energy expenditure, there is some variation in this amount from person to person and even for the same person at different times, depending on his efficiency at the task, the muscular requirements for a particular task, and individual differences in body weight.

Your body uses calories for all physiological functions, both voluntary and involuntary. When you are asleep you utilize an average of 65 calories an hour. As body movements increase, the caloric

This chapter is excerpted with minor modifications from *How to be a good loser: A behavior modification workbook*. Copyright © 1974 by Behavior Associates, 330 E. 13th Street, Tucson, Arizona. Used with permission.

Figure 8-1   Calorie Output Per Activity

When the body is at rest, you use 65 calories an hour.

When you engage in light physical work, you use 175 to 200 calories per hour.

When you engage in moderate exercise, you use 250 to 300 calories per hour.

When you engage in heavy exercise, you use 350 to 400 calories per hour.

Activity	*Calories Expended Per Hour*
Bicycling, moderate speed	175
Carpentry, heavy	161
Dancing	266
Horseback riding, walk	98
Horseback riding, trot	301
Ironing, 5-pound iron	70
Skating	245
Vacuuming	189
Swimming, 2 miles per hour	553
Walking, 3 miles per hour	140
Walking, 4 miles per hour	238
Walking, 5.3 miles per hour	581

output increases. Figure 8-1 (Calorie Output Per Activity) will provide working estimates to help you measure your typical output.

Daily Exercise Record

Record all exercise of any significance on the Daily Exercise Record (figure 8-2). It is not necessary to list sitting, reading, eating, or the usual routine activities of daily living. Should you walk, run, engage in sports or vigorous exercise, keep track of the time spent and the energy expended. Using figure 8-1, classify such activities as light, moderate, or heavy. Since your output will vary with the vigor required to perform a task, you will want to account for these differences.

Figure 8-2 Daily Exercise Record

ACTIVITY	TIME SPENT	CALORIES USED

Your baseline will not reflect your entire level of caloric output but, rather, your present rate of exercise. In a later step you will design a plan to increase the amount of exercise.

Daily Exercise Chart

On your Daily Exercise Chart (figure 8-3) record each day's total energy expenditure. The graph, kept visible, will dramatize your effort and remind you not to let up.

Exercise Contract

Exercise is as much as part of reducing as controlling calories. Overweight people are often comparatively inactive people or people who have become more sedentary with age. The so-called middle-age spread comes with the decline in energy output. You may be eating no more, even less than you formerly did, but still gaining weight. You forget, though, that you are less active and using less energy to perform long-practiced tasks and that a couple of deep knee bends are not going to reduce the bulge of the hips.

Use your Daily Exercise Record to determine how much energy you are expending aside from your basic daily tasks. Burning up 3,500 calories in exercise reduces body weight by a pound. Actually, it makes no difference whether you reduce your food intake by that amount or increase your activity to utilize that number of calories; the weight loss will be the same. Take your choice. However, decreasing intake and increasing output at the same time is the fastest way to a new waistline. Some recent research shows that dieting alone will not cause a sustained weight loss, that exercise must also be a component. Certainly from the standpoint of health, that is clearly the way to reduce. Americans are only now becoming convinced that they are out of shape, out of condition, and out of excuses. Health and exercise clubs have burgeoned all over the country to meet the demands. Joining one is a fine idea if you continue long enough to make the expense worthwhile. Possibly because exercise becomes boring, most people let up after an enthusiastic beginning. Social exercise is more pleasurable than solitary exercise, and you are more likely to continue on a regular basis when you are socially involved.

Whatever exercise you choose, try to make it more vigorous

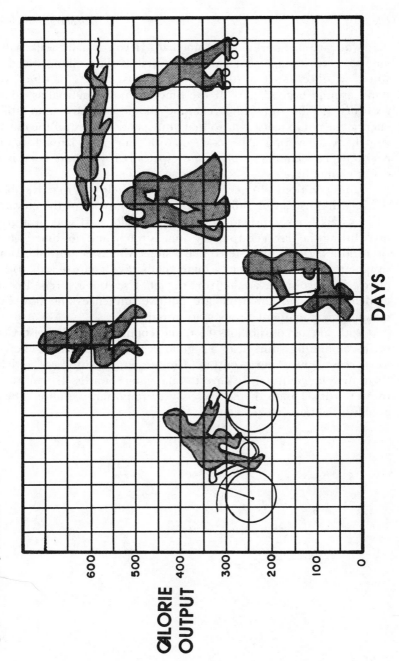

Figure 8-3   Daily Exercise Chart

than you are ordinarily accustomed to. If you usually walk half a mile to work, double that amount as well as the walking speed. If you bowl once a week, add another activity. Sports in which you stand around a good part of the time are not beneficial as calorie reducers. To be significant, exercise should be active and utilize energy but not exhaust you so that you spend the rest of the day on your back recovering. Always check with your physician before embarking on an ambitious program, especially if you have been inactive for some time.

Little additions of energy users will also help you to move about more. Walk instead of riding, use the stairs instead of the elevator, run or walk briskly instead of meandering along. If you sit a great deal during the day, get up every hour, stretch, and do some isometric routines. Don't save steps, make steps whenever possible. Don't sit quietly, move about. Join a hiking club, take a nature walk, ride a bicycle, park your car a mile from the job. Use your Exercise Record to determine who and what are positive influences and how they may help you maintain an exercise program.

With all the possibilities in mind, complete the Exercise Contract, committing yourself to a regular regime of additional exercise to increase your caloric output. Choose your reinforcers and list them in your contract. Be sure to take your rewards. If you tire of the rewards, change them. This is very important because it helps establish the new habits.

Figure 8-4   Exercise Contract

EXERCISE CNTRACT

On _____ I will begin exercising.
I will increase my calorie output by
_____ calories per day.

Each day that I meet this goal I will
reward myself with: _____
_____
_____

Each week that I have met all
seven exercise goals I will reward
myself with: _____
_____
_____

signed: _____
date: _____

part IV

conclusion

9

Clinical Considerations in Behavioral Treatment of Obesity

Edward E. Abramson

Behavior modification is the best treatment for obesity. It is far from being a perfect or even a good treatment. Rather, it excels by virtue of the demonstrated ineffectiveness of other types of treatment. Behavioral self-control is probably the only treatment approach that has been able to demonstrate weight loss with any degree of consistency. The experimental evidence presented in chapter 2 warrants cautious optimism rather than complacency. When you plan to implement a behavioral program, you should be aware of the possible shortcomings as applied to your patients or clients.

One important finding that emerges from the vast majority of experimental studies is that, even in the most effective programs, there is a wide range of response to treatment. The average weight loss of the group may be impressive, but inevitably there are several participants who did not lose weight. At present there is no convincing explanation for this phenomenon. There are, however, several factors independent of the programs themselves which may affect the amount of weight lost by a participant. Most of these contributing factors have not been investigated experimentally. The discussion that follows must, therefore, be considered somewhat speculative.

In my experience treating obese patients, cognitive, affective, and interpersonal factors exert the most influence in determining the ultimate success of treatment. Thinking (cognition) and emotions or feelings (affect) have traditionally been underemphasized by behavior therapists. Recently researchers have started to investigate the effects of cognitive and affective variables on treatment success (e.g., Mahoney 1974). Since most of this research is at an early stage of development, no laws or general principles have been discovered that could be mechanically applied in a weight control program. If, however, you are aware of some of the more common pitfalls, you should be able to help your patients avoid them.

Cognitive Factors

Mahoney and Mahoney (1976*a*) describe three types of maladaptive cognitive behaviors: standard setting, cognitive claustrophobia, and private monologues. Many, if not most, obese people are unrealistic in the standards they set for themselves. The promoters of fad diets and miracle cures are well aware of this tendency and exploit it for all that it is worth with advertisements promising quick and effortless weight loss. The overweight person frequently believes that this is possible. With the best of intentions, he or she will set a weight reduction goal that is impossible to meet. When it becomes apparent that failure is inevitable, the typical response is to give up all attempts to reduce. As therapists we should anticipate our patients' unrealistic expectations and help them set more appropriate goals. For some patients this may be accomplished by a careful explanation of the purpose of the program and the need for permanent habit change rather than quick weight loss. Others may require more individual attention. The therapist should be prepared to explore with patients their goals and the subjective meaning that weight reduction has for them. In terms of the patients' morale and health, it would be better to decide not to participate in the program than to have them continue with unrealistic expectations and ultimately fail.

Realistic goals include weight loss of no more than 1 or 2 pounds per week, calorie consumption of no less than 1,000 calories per day, physical activity and exercise that is consistent with the individual's life-style, and most importantly, allowance for occasional transgressions. Since it is inevitable that there will be a relapse from time to time, the patient should take this into account when setting goals. Setting flexible goals which anticipate the occasional infraction will help prevent what the Mahoneys call cognitive claustrophobia.

As a result of their high standards, obese individuals frequently find themselves in a trap of their own making. Since they have restricted their own behavior in terms of absolutes (e.g., "This is my last milk shake"), they begin to feel claustrophobic. The all-or-none character of their self-imposed standards has the effect of intensifying the desire for the forbidden foods. It is not unusual for a patient to vow total abstinence from a favored food. A period of deprivation has the effect of further enhancing its attractiveness to the point where the patient becomes preoccupied with thoughts of the milk shake or pizza. Inevitably the obese individual succumbs to temptation. This is followed by great relief at the start of the binge and extreme guilt, shame, and depression shortly thereafter. The patient feels that he has failed and there is no value in further efforts. Even when the reaction is less than a full-scale eating binge, I have found that patients will feel that, since they have "cheated," there is no point in pursuing the program for the rest of the day. With this cognitive set, a minor infraction such as eating a doughnut can prevent what would have otherwise been a successful day. The therapist's job is to challenge this all-or-nothing type of thinking. Mahoney and Mahoney (1976a, 1976b) advocate teaching more reasonable self-statements such as "Eating one doughnut doesn't mean I've blown the whole day" or "A person doesn't get fat because of one 'bad' meal or a 'bad' day—or even a 'bad' week; I'm working on a long-range pattern and a few occasional difficulties are not going to throw me" (p. 103). Musante (1976) refers to nonadherence as "unstructured eating" rather than using the more common term *cheating*. Again, the idea is to alter the patients' self-defeating thoughts about their eating behaviors.

The third type of maladaptive cognitive behavior is the negative private monologue. This consists of all the derogatory statements the patient makes to himself about himself. For the typical obese patient, there are many of these private monologues during the course of a day. Most of them are stated in terms of global, vague traits such as

"I am a fat slob" and "I am a failure" (Mahoney and Mahoney 1976*a*). Of course there is no way of proving or disproving these traits. As a result, the negative self-evaluation tends to be relatively permanent. Thus the patient who has adhered to the program for several consecutive days is still a "fat slob" because of earlier unstructured eating. The natural tendency to notice, enjoy, and appreciate one's accomplishments tends to be absent in the area of food consumption. The therapist should help the patient to modify negative monologues. This may be difficult for the nondirective therapist who has been trained to reflect the patient's feelings since the therapist is required to directly challenge the maladaptive cognitions. If necessary, there are several behavioral techniques which will supplement the cognitive reeducation. The patients can be taught to monitor their monologues in the same way that they previously learned to monitor food consumption. Making use of an index card or small diary, the patient can record the date and time of each occurrence, the content of the monologue, and precipitating events or other environmental circumstances. Typically, a pattern will emerge. The therapist can suggest modifications such as engaging in competing activities during periods of high risk.

Another technique, coverant conditioning (Homme 1965), can be used to promote more positive private monologues. This technique is an application of the Premack Principle to one's own thoughts. The Premack Principle holds that low probability behaviors, such as doing homework, can be reinforced with high probability behaviors, such as playing ball. Thus frequently occurring behaviors are made to be contingent upon desirable private monologues such as "I have done a good job today." I used coverant conditioning with an overweight nurse I was treating. Together we prepared several short lists of her strengths and accomplishments. One list was taped to her phone each day. Before making or answering a call she was required to read and repeat to herself one of the statements. She seemed to enjoy the frequent reminder of her strong points and profited from the procedure.

In summary, even the best program is not going to be effective if the patient does not follow it. The various types of cognitive traps described can subvert your efforts. Being aware of their occurrence and helping your patient modify maladaptive cognitions will greatly enhance the effectiveness of treatment.

Affective Factors

The role of emotions in determining the eating behavior of obese people has been stressed by most nonbehavioral theorists. As we have seen in chapter 1, the evidence that eating is precipitated by emotional states is equivocal. The results of treatments aimed at changing the emotional character of obese individuals (i.e., traditional psychotherapy) are unequivocally poor. While our primary emphasis is on the overt behaviors that contribute to obesity, we should not totally ignore the affective states of our patients.

On the most basic physiological level, there is evidence (e.g., Nisbett 1972) that the juvenile onset obese may experience untoward emotional symptoms during and after treatment. The behavioral therapist should be on the lookout for emotional side effects of successful weight reduction, especially toward the end of treatment and during follow-up sessions. While there are no reports in the literature of behavioral treatment of these side effects, systematic desensitization and other behavioral procedures may prove useful. Wolpe (1973) is a good reference for these treatments.

After reviewing the literature, Stunkard and Rush (1974) concluded that "there is a high incidence of symptoms of emotional illness in outpatients treated for obesity" (p. 526). In my experience, depression has been a common complaint among grossly overweight patients. Whether the depression, or other affective disturbance, is the cause of, result of, or unrelated to their obesity is of secondary importance; behavioral treatment will be difficult or impossible while the patient is acutely depressed. The housewife who spends much of her time in bed and feels unable to cope with her family, household chores, and other responsibilities will be unable to monitor her food intake or engage in any of the self-control behaviors required for successful treatment. In several instances, I have found assertive training (Alberti and Emmons 1974) to be helpful. Musante (1976) reports that assertive training is an integral part of the program at Duke University's Dietary Rehabilitation Clinic. Teaching a patient to assert himself serves several purposes. First, patients who typically overeat when in a socially stressful situation will learn more adaptive responses that do not require calorie consumption. Second, assertive training has been successfully used to treat depression (e.g., Lazarus 1971) and other emotional problems. Third, the patient should experience some successes early in treatment as a result of the assertive training. This is particularly important since the ultimate reinforcement for continuing treatment (i.e., weight loss) may not be immediately forthcoming. It is helpful to be able to demonstrate to the patient that he is capable of exerting influence to change his life situation. A final benefit is that assertive training teaches the patient skills that will probably be necessary to change patterns of family interaction that may contribute to the weight problem.

Interpersonal Factors

Eating and exercise do not occur in a vacuum. Frequently the patient's obesity has become a significant factor in his interpersonal relationships. For example, the patient's obesity may be used by the spouse as a weapon in marital conflicts (e.g., "I'll stop drinking when you lose weight"). Stuart (1972) has suggested that obesity can serve the function of a chastity belt. To the extent that the wife is overweight and unattractive, the insecure husband feels safe from competition for her affections. In this type of situation, family members may reinforce the patient's inappropriate eating patterns in order to avoid having to change their own behavior. Even in the best of marriages however, family members may have come to doubt the patient's ability to lose weight because of the numerous unsuccessful attempts to diet. As a result, family members may nag the patient or disparage his efforts. Also, family members may object when the patient tries to alter established eating routines or removes favorite high-calorie foods from the house.

Passive acceptance of the program by family members is a bare minimum if treatment is to be successful. Typically, behavioral programs have focused exclusively on the obese individual. McReynolds (1975) feels that this "one man, one fork" doctrine ignores the vital interpersonal aspects of eating and weight reduction. He advocates the behavioral treatment of the family since most people eat and live with others; family therapy is more efficient if there is more than one obese person, and involving several people makes it more likely that there will be early detection and hopefully prevention of obesity in the children. The last consideration is especially important because of the likelihood of critical periods during childhood when excessive calorie consumption can lead to irreversible increases in the number of fat cells. Family treatment may help avoid future generations of juvenile onset obesity. The preliminary results of

McReynolds's study suggest that husband-wife and father-son treatment pairs are successful while the treatment of mother and daughter together presents problems.

Even if there is only one obese person in the family, participation and support of the others should be enlisted. Ferguson (1976) indicates that the Stanford Eating Disorders Clinic reviews the program with the spouse and requires that he or she be available to assist with some phases of treatment. In my clinical work I routinely invite the spouse and other family members to participate. After an explanation of the goals and methods of treatment, I request that they help by praising appropriate behaviors rather than criticizing or nagging the patient about unstructured eating or failure to exercise. They can also help by buying and preparing low-calorie foods, avoiding social pressure to eat and by being available to participate in alternative activities when the patient feels compelled to eat. If assertive training is part of the program, I will ask the spouse to attend several sessions to help in the rehearsal of new responses, so that he or she understands and is prepared for the change in interpersonal behavior. Although the usefulness of family involvement has not yet been demonstrated experimentally, Mahoney (1973) found a significant correlation ($r=.69$) between a measure of family support and patient weight loss.

Occasionally the emotional or other disturbance of potential patients may be serious enough to exclude them from treatment. Many ongoing treatment facilities routinely screen out psychotic applicants. It might also be worthwhile to assess the life situation of the applicant. Jeffrey (in press) proposed several questions that can be used to assess the appropriateness of treatment: (1) Does the patient have good, long-term reasons for desiring weight loss? (2) Are significant others (e.g., husband, parents) willing to help? and, (3) Is there enough stability in the patient's life so that he can devote the necessary time and effort to changing his or her eating patterns? If the patient cannot make the commitment required, or if the life situation is such that he would not be able to follow through, it would probably be wise to postpone treatment.

Therapist Effectiveness

The role of the therapist and therapist characteristics necessary for successful treatment are debatable issues at present. The studies of bibliotherapy, reviewed in chapter 2, suggest that the therapist may not be necessary for effective treatment. The implication of these findings is that the principles and techniques used in these programs are powerful in themselves; the human component in their application is not necessary. Wollersheim (1970), Abrahms and Allen (1974), Balch and Balch (in press), Lindstrom, Balch, and Reese (1975) among others have failed to find differences between therapists conducting similar treatments. Again, this suggests that the behavioral techniques are sufficiently robust so that specific therapeutic skill is not required in their application. While it would be nice if we had a treatment so effective that it could be applied by anyone with or without training, I think that this is not the case. Only one of the eight studies cited above did not use college students as subjects. Franzini and Grimes (1976) point out that participants who are not college students being paid or receiving credit for participating in a professor's study are less likely to respond to the implicit demand characteristics of the situation and less likely to be enthusiastic about techniques requiring time and effort from them. My hunch is that the therapist's skills would be required to keep up the interest and participation of older patients who are not college students. Since the college subjects are likely to be more responsive, differences in skill between therapists would have less of an impact on treatment outcome for this group.

Several recent studies have demonstrated differences between therapists in their effectiveness although the variables which determine these differences are still a matter for speculation. Levitz and Stunkard (1974), using ongoing TOPS (Take Off Pounds Sensibly) groups, compared the effectiveness of behavior modification conducted by mental health professionals (psychiatric residents or graduate students in clinical psychology) with that of an identical program led by trained TOPS chapter leaders. The professionally led groups lost more weight at the end of treatment. The difference was even more striking at the one-year follow-up. Weight loss was slightly greater for participants in the professionally led groups while those in the groups led by the TOPS leaders regained virtually all the weight that had been lost. Both groups were superior to comparable groups which followed the regular TOPS routine. Ferguson (1976) reported differences in outcome between groups led by different therapists. He lists leadership style, leader interest in the program, and the leader's previous experience with the program as some of the factors contributing to the differences in therapeutic effectiveness. He concluded that the differences were so great that nonspecific variables may be more important than the behavior modification techniques themselves. In view of the considerable literature demonstrating the ineffectiveness of traditional psychotherapy regardless of the therapists' skills, it would be difficult to endorse the view that therapist skill is more important than the behavioral techniques. Nonetheless, there appears to be evidence that some level of therapeutic skill is required for successful implementation of behavioral programs, at least with noncollegiate patients.

The nature of the therapeutic attributes required remains ill defined. Jeffrey (in press) suggests that, in addition to knowledge of behavior modification principles, the therapist must have basic interviewing and interpersonal skills and be sensitive to the patient's needs. In supervising graduate students in counseling psychology, I have found that patient weight loss in a behavioral group treatment was related to measures of counselor effectiveness (Carkhuff 1969). One of the graduate students, a thin male who was somewhat skeptical of the behavioral procedures, was less successful (i.e., had less weight loss and a greater attrition rate) in treating overweight college women than a female graduate student using exactly the same procedures. She had previously had some problems with weight control and was enthusiastic about the program. Clearly, the issue of therapist characteristics affecting treatment outcome requires further research. When the critical variables are isolated, it should be possible to select or train therapists to maximize treatment effectiveness.

Individualizing Treatment

The programs in chapter 3 and 4 of this book present a wide variety of behavioral techniques. Implicit in many of the techniques is the idea that obesity is a unitary disorder characterized by an obese eating style which has been learned (Mahoney 1975*a*). Hagen (1976) suggests that there may be several types of obesity with differing etiologies. If this position is correct, it would be reasonable to assume that any one technique need not be equally useful for all obese people. Mahoney and Mahoney (1976*c*) found that some of their patients have profited from stimulus control techniques while others reported that self-reward was more beneficial. Unfortunately there is no scheme currently available for matching techniques to patients. In chapter 4 Wollersheim suggests that patients try all of the techniques presented but continue to use only those that are effective for them.

In the absence of firm guidelines for individualizing treatment, I would like to offer some tentative suggestions. Occasionally the therapist will be confronted with an obese patient who does not seem to be eating excessively. If after reviewing the Eating Diary, probing for instances of unrecorded eating, checking with family members, and waiting several weeks, the therapist is convinced that the patient is not eating excessively, the focus of treatment should be altered to stress the exercise components. Obviously there is little point in teaching stimulus control exercises when the patient consumes fewer than 1,000 calories per day. The techniques presented in chapter 8 should be the primary component of treatment.

Even in the majority of cases where overeating plays a crucial role in the development and maintenance of obesity, the therapist may want to emphasize one or two of the techniques presented. Usually the "Circumstances" column in the Eating Diary form will indicate specific problem areas for the patient which will enable the therapist to select the appropriate technique. For example, if the Diary indicates that eating takes place in many different environments, the therapist probably should concentrate on helping the client limit eating to a single situation. On the other hand, if the Diary shows large amounts of food consumed at infrequent meals, it would be preferable to concentrate on those exercises that slow the rate of food consumption.

A final issue is the degree to which treatment should be individualized in order to deal with affective disturbances and other personal problems mentioned earlier. At present, it is not clear to what extent this is desirable. Some investigators (e.g., Balch and Ross 1974) have stated explicitly that their treatment sessions were conducted solely in a lecture format. Others have been vague in terms of specifying the way in which treatment was presented. Programs encouraging group discussion would be more likely to elicit personal concerns not directly related to weight. Although there is no research on this topic, discussion of personal problems would be acceptable and probably useful in individual sessions. In group treatment, however, there may not be sufficient time to deal with concerns unrelated to weight. Until clear guidelines are available, the therapist will have to decide which type of question or discussion is inappropriate and then use his leadership skills to limit discussion without offending participants.

In summary, the various behavioral programs should not be viewed as cookbooks containing the perfect recipe for treatment. Although each of the programs in this book is among the best of its type, they all reflect the current state of the art. The necessity for a discussion of nonspecific factors is an indication of the deficiencies in behavioral treatment of obesity. Future progress will require: (1) the development of new techniques and the refinement of current procedures, and (2) the expansion of behavioral programs to include in a systematic fashion the cognitive, affective, interpersonal, and other variables that have been roughly described in this chapter. When this has been accomplished, we will have a truly effective technology of weight control.

appendixes

APPENDIX A
Weight Reduction Program
Questionnaire

1. NAME: _____

   ADDRESS: _____

   PHONE: _____ AGE: _____ SEX: _____

2. How did you hear about the weight reduction program:

   a. Friend _____   d. Chronicle Ad _____
   b. Referral _____   e. Other _____
   c. Posters _____

3. a. What is your height? _____
   b. What is your present weight? _____ (weigh in)
   c. How long have you been your present weight? _____

4. Have you participated in any type of weight program before?

   Yes _____   No _____

   If yes, where _____

           what program _____

           what happened _____

5. Have you talked to a physician before about your weight?

   Yes _____   No _____

   If yes, what were his recommendations: _____
   _____
   _____
   _____

6. a. How many pounds do you want to lose? _____
   b. What is your ideal weight? _____

7. Why do you want to lose weight? _____
   _____
   _____
   _____

147

8. What do you feel have been the causes of your over weight? _____
    _____
    _____
    _____
    _____

(PLEASE PLACE AN X AT THE POINT ON THE LINE WHICH MOST APPROXIMATES WHERE YOU ARE)

9. How much control do you feel <u>you</u> have in losing weight?

    no control   total control

10. How committed are you to losing weight?

    no commitment   total commitment

11. How ready are you to participate now in the weight reduction program at the Counseling Center.

    not ready   completely ready

12. How much responsibility do you feel <u>you</u> have for losing weight?

    none   total

13. How motivated are you to lose weight?

    very little   extremely motivated

14. Rate how much you would like to receive congratulations for losing weight from each of the following.

    a. spouse

    none   very much

    b. male parent

    none   very much

    c. female parent

    none   very much

    d. boyfriend

    none   very much

    e. girlfriend

    none   very much

    f. siblings

    none   very much

g. no one

| none | | | | | | | | very much |

h. other _____

| none | | | | | | | | very much |

i. myself

| none | | | | | | | | very much |

15. Which of the following months will you be in Salt Lake City.

March_____   May_____   July_____

April_____   June_____   August_____

APPENDIX B
Weight Reduction Program
Behavioral Contract

This agreement, made and entered into this _____ day of _____

197___, by and between _____ party of the

first part, and _____ party of the second

part, witnesseth:

Said party of the first part agrees to work diligently in losing weight. To

insure this, the party of the first part will seek to lose _____ to

_____ pounds each week. Said party will attempt to obtain and maintain

the desired weight of _____ pounds.

The party of the first part agrees to do the following:

    (1)   To daily graph his weight and bring his graph to each session.

    (2)   To read his statements of consequences for losing or not losing

           weight at the following times and places.

	Time	Place
a.		
b.		
c.		

    (3)   To participate in a weekly exercise program.

           a.   What exercises _____

           b.   Where _____

           c.   When _____

    (4)   The party of the first part agrees to actively institute the stimulus

           control techniques as prescribed by himself and the party of the second

           part.

    (5)   The party of the first part further agrees to reduce caloric intake

           and alter caloric intake patterns as defined from information on the

           Eating Diary.

(6)   The party of the first party agrees to deposit a total amount of

_____ to the Weight Program. The party of the second part

agrees to pay back a proportion _____ each week to be

earned on the following basis.

                                %   Weekly Total   Amount Earned

(1) Attendance ____25%____ X _____ = _____

(2) Bring completed weekly graph to each meeting.

                  ____25%____ X _____ = _____

(3) Lose between _____ and _____ pounds

                  ____50%____ X _____ = _____

                              Total possible = _____
                              Weekly Earnings

(7)   The party of the first part agrees that the total amount remaining

in his deposit will be forfeited to the weight control program if

he drops out of said program without first having a private interview

with the party of the second part.

(8)   Other objectives

In consideration for all of the above, the party of the second part agrees
to examine diligently all graphs and materials prepared by the party of the
first part, agrees to examine the weight of the party of the first part on a
regular and defined basis (i.e., twice weekly) and further acknowledges that
he will praise the party of the first part whenever a reduction of weight occurs
and otherwise encourage the party of the first part.

In witness thereof both parties have hereunto set their hands and seals
the day and year above written.

_____   _____
Witness   Party of the first part

_____   _____
Date   Party of the second part

APPENDIX C
Daily Weight Graph

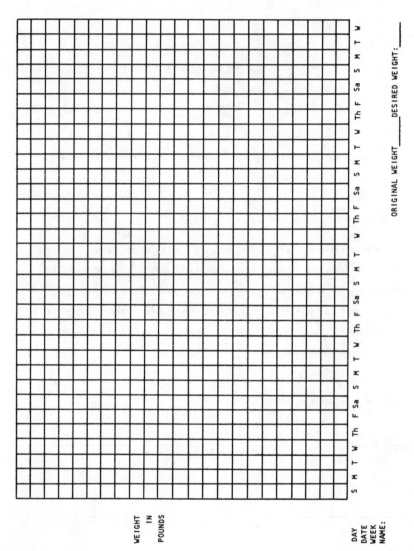

WEIGHT IN POUNDS

DAY
DATE
WEEK
NAME:

ORIGINAL WEIGHT_____ DESIRED WEIGHT:_____

APPENDIX D
Sample Weekly Weight Graph

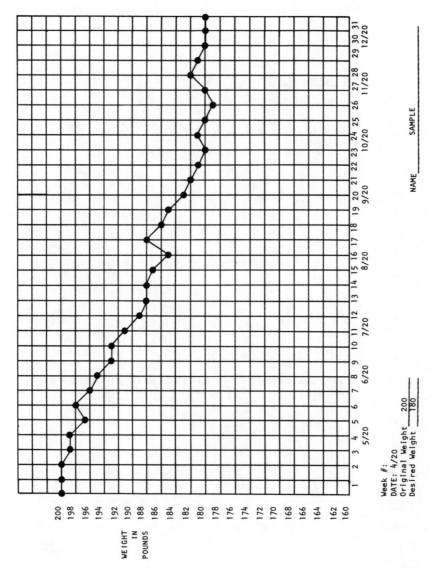

153

APPENDIX E
Reinforcement Menu

Your reasons for losing weight

A. Negative reasons (consequences) for not losing weight.

1. I'll lose my money deposited with the weight loss program.
2. I'll have a greater probability of having more ilnesses and dying of a heart attack.
3. I won't be able to fit into my smaller clothes.

4.

5.

6.

7.

8.

9.

10.

.

.

B. Positive reasons (consequences) for losing weight.

1. I will earn back my money I deposited with the weight reduction program.
2. I will be less prone to get illnesses and die of a heart attack.
3. I will look and feel slimmer.

4.

5.

6.

7.

8.

9.

10.

154

APPENDIX F
Physician Permission Form

UNIVERSITY OF UTAH
COUNSELING CENTER

WEIGHT REDUCTION PROGRAM

Mr./Mrs./Miss _____ is planning to

participate in the Counseling Center's behavioral modification program for

gradual and controlled weight reduction. I have examined Mr./Mrs./Miss

_____ and have _____/have not _____

found him/her in sufficiently good health at this time to participate in such

a program.

In addition, I have discussed with him/her the amount of weekly weight loss

that would be best for him and have suggested a diet.

_____
(Sign)

_____
(Date)

APPENDIX G
Eating Diary

Name _____

Date _____

Time	Antecedent Event (Place, Situation before and while eating)	Eating Responses (Kind & Amount of Food Eaten)				Subsequent Events (Events following eating)
		Kind	Amount	Calories	Cumulative Calories	
Breakfast						
Morning Snack						
Lunch						
Afternoon Snack						
Dinner						
Evening Snack						
Total						

APPENDIX H
Instructions for
Computing Average
Daily Caloric Intake

1. Find the number of calories in each item of food consumed during the baseline period. (A calorie counter booklet, which can be purchased in a supermarket, is essential for this process.)
2. Total the caloric intake for each of the six eating time periods for each day.
3. Add the daily totals for each eating time period and divide each of these totals by the number of days. The result is the average daily caloric intake for each of the eating time periods.

These figures will help in the assessment of average daily eating patterns.

The weekly eating patterns can be assessed by merely obtaining the total caloric intake for each day in the baseline phase and then comparing these totals.

APPENDIX I
Illustrative Case Histories

Case 1: A Multiple Intervention

Jolene came in desiring to lose weight to "improve physical appearance and thereby improve confidence in dating." She initially wanted to lose 22 pounds, attaining a final weight of 120 pounds. As the causes for being overweight, she listed: (1) "anxiety involved with dating (about getting seriously involved)," (2) "sometimes school or anger tension (rare)." Control of her anxiety and tension were stated as an additional goal which she also desired to attain. Jolene was referred to a therapist to meet that goal and was also concurrently included in the weight reduction program.

For the first ten weeks of the program her weight loss and attendance records were the best of anyone in her group. She cooperated very well in carrying out the tasks given her and met her weight loss goal every week but one. However, during the private weigh-ins with the weight reduction therapist, she expressed anxiety about "getting under 130 pounds" because she would then become "more attractive to boys." According to the other therapist helping her with the control of her anxiety, getting below 130 pounds was frightening because of the increased potential of sexual involvement.

On the eleventh week of treatment Jolene asked the weight reduction therapist not to tell her the exact weight she had attained but to write it down on her graph so that her mother could keep

---

The patient's names in each of these case histories are pseudonyms used to assure confidentiality.

track. Jolene said that this way she would not know when she weighed below 130 pounds. On the fifteeth week at 127 pounds she came in anxious and upset, saying she would have to quit the program. Instead, it was decided that she would begin on the maintenance portion of the program and attempt to keep her weight at or below 132 pounds. Jolene felt she had failed in the program, so the therapist helped her to see that she had done fairly well. She maintained her weight below 132 pounds for three months, after which she terminated the weight program, remaining in therapy working on her other goals.

Case 2: Competing Reinforcement

Judy was a twenty-year-old single female who lived with her parents. Her weight at the beginning of the program was 139 pounds. From the outset she showed approach-avoidance behavior concerning the program. Statements like "I don't know if I'll be here next time," or "Are you sure this program really works?" were typical of Judy. She was more than fifteen minutes late to three of the first five 45-minute weekly sessions. After the fifth week her attendance became sporadic and irregular. At the sessions attended, she did not bring her weight graphs and other self-monitoring materials. During the eighth week of treatment she came in for a private interview. During the interview she reported being under stress from school and her job. She also mentioned that her parents were "upset" with her because she had moved away from home to live with some friends. Her parents had told her it was "unheard of" in the "old country" for a daughter to move out before marriage. Also, during the course of the interview Judy stated that her mother did not want her to lose weight because in the "old country" it was normal to eat lots of food and get fat. Judy said she would attempt to continue to lose weight now that she had moved.

In the tenth week of treatment she came in and said that she wanted to drop out because the meeting times interfered with her job and that she was under stress at work. Her weight was 138 pounds at termination. In ten weeks she was called in for a follow-up. She had gone to a popular commercial weight control program four times. Her weight was 137 pounds. She was referred for additional counseling.

Case 3: Money as a Reinforcer

Susan was middle-aged, single, and divorced, with a reported history of excessive weight for a period of five years. At the beginning of the treatment procedures she weighed 154 pounds. Her stated reasons for wanting to lose weight were to "look better" and "feel better." Data on her eating patterns showed that she overate most often when she became bored or lonely. She reported having been able to lose up to 20 pounds during a self-imposed diet. However, she had been able to maintain this loss for only a brief period. She set as her initial goal a weight loss of 21 pounds. On a self-report item asking how much responsibility she felt for her weight loss, she rated herself at six on a seven-point scale. She rated herself at seven on the same scale in her commitment to lose weight. During treatment she had marked success and was able to lose at least 1 pound each of the twenty-four weeks with only four exceptions. At the end of the treatment phase she had achieved a weight loss of 24 pounds. At six months, after the end of regular treatment sessions, she made two statements that were characteristic of her response to the treatment approach: "Money was a good reinforcer for me," and "I managed to really control my eating habits at first because of the contract but later because I desired to." At this final meeting her weight was 134 pounds.

Case 4: Boosters during Maintenance

Jack was a married male who had a history of excessive weight for five previous years. At the beginning of the program he weighed 200 pounds. He reported that he had made no attempt to lose weight in the past. He specified a long-term weight loss of 30 pounds as his goal. As reasons for wanting to lose weight, he indicated a desire for "better health, better looks, and increased agility in the handball court." He recognized that his overweight condition was a function of "poor eating habits," which he defined as "eating too much of the wrong food at the wrong time." On a scale from one to seven, he graded himself at seven in terms of commitment to weight loss. Jack was very successful in treatment. He accomplished the monitoring tasks regularly, and lost weight regularly. His weight was 170 pounds at the end of treatment.

During the maintenance phase of the program, Jack experienced difficulty maintaining his new eating habits. As a result, he contacted the therapist for related booster sessions. There were three booster sessions. These were 10-minute meetings where he weighed-in and stated his maintenance goals and his strategy for stabilizing eating habits. During these sessions the therapist reinforced appropriate behaviors and eating strategies. No monetary contingencies were used in these sessions. At six months after treatment, his weight was 172 pounds.

Case 5: Energy Expenditure and Intervening Problems

Dick was thirty years old, married, and had one child. He had been overweight since high school. For some time he had wanted to lose 20 pounds (from 200 to 180 pounds). Initially he attended the weight program regularly, involved himself in a vigorous athletic program as specified in his behavioral contract. He lost over 15 pounds. Dick enjoyed sports, and his active participation in an exercise and sports program substantially increased his energy expenditure. He also cut down his caloric intake, particularly by reducing between-meal snacks. Both self-report and therapist observations confirmed that a major factor in Dick's weight loss was the substantial increase in his energy output.

Starting with the fifteenth week Dick missed several of the weekly sessions. The therapist contacted him to find out if anything was wrong. A subsequent personal interview indicated that he was having marital difficulties and that he and his wife were seeing a marriage counselor. It was mutually agreed between Dick and the weight control therapist that his weight contract should be suspended until he could work out his marital problems. A subsequent interview revealed that Dick and his wife had decided to get divorced. Because of this fact, that Dick was making a readjustment in his life, he and the therapist mutually agreed to terminate the weight contract.

Dick had marital problems and was seeing a marriage counselor before he started the weight program. Even with the stresses on Dick, he was able to maintain his weight 10 pounds or more below what it was at the beginning of the program.

Case 6: The Use of Stimulus Objects as Reminders

Linda, a twenty-three-year-old married secretary, had a weight loss goal of 30 pounds, from 140 to 110. She used various high-protein diets to lose the first 20 pounds over a twelve-week period, but then hit a plateau which persisted for the next nine weeks. Linda had a picture of herself in a bikini at 140 pounds which she taped to the refrigerator door. Later she taped to the refrigerator a second ("after") photo of herself in a new bikini to help her maintain the loss. During the difficult plateau period she increased her activity level by walking and bike-riding daily. She also maintained a low-calorie but varied diet. Linda kept her list of reasons for wanting to lose weight taped to the closet door where she kept her scale. She found that the positive list of reasons to lose weight was much more effective for her than the negative list of bad things about being overweight. She reached her weight goal during the course of the program but felt better and had more energy at 115 pounds. She then renegotiated her goal weight to 115 pounds.

Our thanks and appreciation to Carol Atkinson for providing case history 6.

References

Abrahms, J. L., and Allen, G. J. 1974. Comparative effectiveness of situational programming, financial pay-offs and group pressure in weight reduction. *Behav. Therapy* 5:391–400.

Abramson, E. E. 1973. A review of behavioral approaches to weight control. *Behav. Res. & Therapy* 11:547–56.

Abramson, E. E., and Stinson, S. G. Boredom and eating in obese and normals. *Addict. Behav.*, in press.

Abramson, E. E., and Wunderlich, R. A. 1972. Anxiety, fear and eating: A test of the psychosomatic concept of obesity. *J. Abnorm. Psychol.* 79:317–21.

Alberti, R. E., and Emmons, M. L. 1974. *Your perfect right.* 2d ed. San Luis Obispo, Ca.: Impact.

Aragona, J.; Cassady, J.; and Drabman, R. S. 1975. Treating overweight children through parental training and contingency contracting. *J. Appl. Behav. Anal.* 8:269–78.

Ashem, B., and Donner, L. 1968. Covert sensitization with alchoholics: A controlled replication. *Behav. Res. & Therapy* 6:7–12.

Ashem, B.; Poser, E.; and Trudall, P. 1970. The use of covert sensitization in the treatment of overeating. Paper presented at the Association for the Advancement of Behavior Therapy, Miami, September 1970.

Ayllon, T. 1963. Intensive treatment of psychotic behaviour by stimulus satiation and food reinforcement. *Behav. Res. & Therapy* 1:53–61.

Baer, D. M.; Wolf, M. M.; and Risley, T. R. 1968. Some current dimensions of applied behavior analysis. *J. Appl. Behav. Anal.* 1:91–7.

Balch, P., and Balch, K. Establishing a campus-wide behavioral weight reduction program through a university student health service: The use and training of health service personnel as behavioral weight therapists. *J. Am. Coll. Health Assoc.,* in press.

Balch, P., and Ross, A. W. 1972. A behaviorally oriented didactic-group treatment of obesity: An exploration study. *J. Behav. Therapy & Exp. Psychiat.* 5:239–43.

———. 1975. Predicting success in weight reduction as a function of locus of control: A unidimensional and multidimensional approach. *J. Consult. Clin. Psychol.* 43:119.

Barlow, D. H.; Leitenberg, H.; and Agras, W. S. 1969. Experimental control of sexual deviation through manipulation of the noxious scene in covert sensitization. *J. Abnorm. Psychol.* 5:596–601.

Bates, M. M., and Johnson, C. D. 1972. *Group leadership: A manual for group counseling leaders.* Denver: Love.

Behnke, A. R.; Osserman, E. F.; and Welham, W. C. 1953. Lean body mass. *Archs. Intern. Med.* 91:585.

Bellack, A. S. 1975. Behavior therapy for weight reduction. *Addict. Behav.* 1:73–82.

———. 1976. A comparison of self-reinforcement and self-monitoring in a weight reduction program. *Behav. Therapy* 7:68–75.

Bellack, A. S., and Rozensky, R. H. 1975. The selection of dependent variables for weight reduction studies. *J. Behav. Therapy & Exp. Psychiat.* 6:83–4.

Bellack, A. S.; Rozensky, R.; and Schwartz, J. 1974. A comparison of two forms of self-monitoring in a behavioral weight reduction program. *Behav. Therapy* 5:523–30.

Bellack, A. S.; Schwartz, J.; and Rozensky, R. H. 1974. The contribution of external control to self-control in a weight reduction program. *J. Behav. Therapy & Exp. Psychiat.* 5:245–50.

Berblinger, K. W. 1969. Obesity and psychologic stress. In *Obesity,* ed. N. L. Wilson. Philadelphia: F. A. Davis.

Bernard, J. L. 1968. Rapid treatment of gross obesity by operant techniques. *Psychol. Rep.* 23:663–68.

Borden, B. L. 1974. Variables relating to success in the behavioral treatment of obesity. Paper presented at the annual meeting, Western Psychological Association, San Francisco, April 1974.

Bradfield, R. B., and Jourdan, M. 1972. Energy expenditure of obese women during weight loss. *Am. J. Clin. Nutr.* 25:971–75.

Bruch, H. 1973. *Eating disorders: Obesity, anorexia nervosa, and the person within.* New York: Basic Books.

Bruch, H., and Waters, I. 1942. Benzedrine sulfate (amphetamine) in the treatment of obese children and adolescents. *J. Pediat.* 20:54–64.

Brunn, A. C., and Hedberg, A. G. 1974. Covert positive reinforcement as a treatment procedure for obesity. *J. Community Psychol.* 2:117–119.

Cappon, D. 1973. *Eating, loving and dying: A psychology of appetites.* Toronto: University of Toronto Press.

Carkhuff, R. R. 1969. *Helping and human relations.* Vol. 2 *Practice and research.* New York: Holt, Rinehart & Winston.

Cautela, J. R. 1966. Treatment of compulsive behavior by covert sensitization. *Psychol. Rec.* 16:33–41.

———. 1967. Covert sensitization. *Psychol. Rep.* 20:459–68.

———. 1968. Behavior therapy and need for behavioral assessment. *Psychotherapy: Theory, Research and Practice* 5:175–79.

———. 1969. Behavior therapy and self-control: Techniques and implications. In *Behavior Therapy: Appraisal and Status,* ed. C. Franks, pp. 323–40. New York: McGraw-Hill.

———. 1970. Covert reinforcement. *Behav. Therapy* 1:33–50.

Cautela, J. R., and Kastenbaum, R. 1967. A reinforcement survey schedule for use in therapy and research. *Psychol. Rep.* 20:115–30.

Cautela, J. R.; Steffan, J.; and Wish, P. An experimental test of covert reinforcement. *J. Clin. & Consult. Psychol.,* in press.

Cautela, J. R.; Walsh, K.; and Wish, P. 1971. The use of covert reinforcement to modify attitudes toward the mentally retarded. *J. Psychol.* 77:257–60.

Chlouverakis, C. 1975. Dietary and medical treatments of obesity: An evaluative review. *Addict. Behav.* 1:3–21.

Christensen, A., and Barrios, E. 1975. Partners, payoffs, and pounds: A treatment program for the overweight. Paper presented at the annual meeting of the Western Psychological Association, Sacramento, California, April 1975.

Craig, L. S. 1969. Anthropometric determinants of obesity. In *Obesity*, ed. N. L. Wilson. Philadelphia: F. A. Davis.

Demke, E. 1971. Effects of taste on the eating behavior of obese and normal persons. Cited in S. Schachter, *Emotion, Obesity and Crime*. New York: Academic Press.

Diament, C., and Wison, G. T. 1975. An experimental investigation of the effects of covert sensitization in an analogue eating situation. *Behav. Therapy* 6:499–509.

Dinoff, M.; Rickard, H. C.; and Colwick, J. 1972. Weight reduction through successive contracts. *Am. J. Orthopsychiat.* 42:110–13.

Drenick, E. J. 1969. Starvation in the management of obesity. In *Obesity*, ed. N. L. Wilson. Philadelphia: F. A. Davis.

Elliott, C. H., and Denney, D. R. 1975. Weight control through covert sensitization and false feedback. *J. Consult. Clin. Psychol.* 42:842–50.

Feinstein, A. R. 1959. The measurement of success in weight reduction. *J. Chron. Dis.* 10:439–56.

Ferguson, J. M. 1976. A clinical program for the behavioral control of obesity. In *Obesity: Behavioral approaches to dietary management*, ed. B. J. Williams, S. Martin, and J. P. Foreyt. New York: Brunner/Mazel.

Ferster, C. B.; Nurnberger, J. I.; and Levitt, E. B. 1962. The control of eating. *J. Mathetics* 1:87–109.

Flannery, R. An investigation of differential effectiveness of office vs. *in vivo* therapy of a simple phobia; an outcome study. *Behav. Therapy & Exp. Psychiat.*, in press.

Food and Drug Administration. 1973. New restrictions on diet pills. *F.D.A. Consumer*, April 1973.

Foreyt, J. P., and Hagen, R. L. 1973. Covert sensitization: Conditioning or suggestion? *J. Abnorm. Psychol.* 82:17–23.

Foreyt, J. P., and Kennedy, W. A. 1971. Treatment of overweight by aversion therapy. *Behav. Res. & Therapy* 9:29–34.

Fowler, R. S.; Fordyce, W. E.; Boyd, V. D.; and Masock, A. J. 1972. The mouthful diet: A behavioral approach to overeating. *Rehab. Psychol.* 19:98–106.

Franks, C. 1967. Reflections upon the treatment of sexual disorders by the behavioral clinicians: An historical comparison with the treatment of the alcoholic. *J. Sex Res.* 3:212–22.

Franzini, L. R., and Grimes, W. B. 1975. Contracting, Stuart's three-dimensional treatment, and a new criterion of change in behavior therapy of the obese. Paper presented at the annual meeting of the Association for Advancement of Behavior Therapy, San Francisco, December 1975.

――――. 1976*a*. Skinfold measures as the criterion of change in weight control studies. *Behav. Therapy* 7:256–60.

――――. 1976*b*. Special treatment strategies for clinicians conducting weight control programs. Paper presented at the annual meeting of the Western Psychological Association, Los Angeles, April 1976.

Gaul, D. J.; Craighead, W. E.; and Mahoney, M. J. 1975. The relationship between eating rates and obesity. *J. Consult. and Clin. Psychol.* 43:123–25.

Glucksman, M. L., and Hirsch, J. 1968. The response of obese patients to weight reduction: A clinical evaluation of behavior. *Psychosom. Med.* 30:1–11.

Glucksman, M. L.; Hirsch, J.; McCully, R. S.; Barron, B. A.; and Knittle, J. L. 1968. The response of obese patients to weight reduction: II. A quantative evaluation of behavior. *Psychosom. Med.* 30:359–73.

Goldiamond, I. 1965. Self-control procedures in personal behavior problems. *Psychol. Rep.* 17:851–68.

Grinker, J.; Hirsch, J.; and Levin, B. 1973. The affective responses of obese patients to weight reduction: A differentiation based on age and onset of obesity. *Psychom. Med.* 35:57–63.

Hagen, R. L. 1974. Group therapy versus bibliotherapy in weight reduction. *Behav. Therapy* 5:222–34.

――――. 1976. Theories of obesity: Is there any hope for order? In *Obesity: Behavioral approaches to dietary management,* ed. B. J. Williams, S. Martin, and J. P. Foreyt. New York: Brunner/Mazel.

Hall, R. G. 1974. Follow up strategies and therapist change in the behavioral treatment of overweight. Paper presented at the annual meeting, Western Psychological Association, San Francisco, April 1974.

Hall, S. M. 1972. Self-control and therapist control in the behavioral treatment of overweight women. *Behav. Res. & Therapy* 10:59–68.

――――. 1973. Behavioral treatment of obesity: A two-year follow-up. *Behav. Res. & Therapy* 11:647–48.

Hall, S. M.; Hall, R. G.; Hanson, R. W.; and Borden, B. L. 1974. Permanence of two self-managed treatments of overweight in university and community populations. *J. Consult. Clin. Psychol.* 42:781–86.

Hanson, R. W. 1974. Effects of programmed learning and therapist-group contact in treating obesity. Paper presented at the annual meeting, Western Psychological Association, San Francisco, California, April 1974.

Harmatz, M. G., and Lapuc, P. 1968. Behavior modification of overeating in a psychiatric population. *J. Consult. Clin. Psychol.* 32:583–87.

Harris, M. B. 1969. Self-directed program for weight control: Pilot study. *J. Abnorm. Psychol.* 74:263–70.

Harris, M. B., and Bruner, C. G. 1971. A comparison of self-control and a contract procedure for weight control. *Behav. Res. & Therapy* 9:347–52.

Harris, M. B., and Hallbauer, E. S. 1973. Self-directed weight control through eating and exercise. *Behav. Res. & Therapy* 11:523–29.

Henley, R. E. 1976. Predicting successful weight loss in humans. Unpublished M.A. thesis, California State University, Chico.

Hirsch, J., and Knittle, J. L. 1970. Cellularity of obese and non-obese adipose tissue. *Fed. Proc.* 29:1516–21.

Holland, J.; Masling, J.; and Copley, D. 1970. Mental illness in lower class normal, obese, and hyperobese women. *Psychosom. Med.* 32:351–57.

Holt, H., and Winick, C. 1961. Group psychotherapy with obese women. *Archs. Gen. Psychiat.* 5:64–76.

Homme, L. E. Perspectives in psychology: xxiv, Control of coverants, the operants of the mind. *Psychol. Rec.* 15:501–11.

Horan, J. J.; Baker, S. B.; Hoffman, A. M.; and Shute, R. E. 1975. Weight loss through variations in the coverant control paradigm. *J. Consult. Clin. Psychol.* 43:68–72.

Horan, J. J., and Johnson, R. G. 1971. Coverant conditioning through a self-management application of the Premack Principle: Its effect on weight reduction. *J. Behav. Therapy & Exp. Psychiat.* 2:243–49.

Hull, C. 1952. *A behavior system.* New Haven: Yale University Press.

Jacobson, E. 1938. *Progressive relaxation.* Chicago: University of Chicago Press.

Janda, L. H., and Rimm, D. C. 1972. Covert sensitization in the treatment of obesity. *J. Abnorm. Psychol.* 80:37–42.

Jeffrey, D. B. 1974. A comparison of the effects of external control and self-control on the modification and maintenance of weight. *J. Abnorm. Psychol.* 83:404–10.

———. 1975*a*. Treatment evaluation issues in research on addictive behaviors. *Addict. Behav.* 1:23–36.

———. 1975*b*. Self-control versus external-control in the modification and maintenance of weight loss. In *Applications of behavior therapy to health care*, ed. R. C. Katz and S. I. Zlutnick. New York: Pergamon.

———. Behavioral management of obesity: Learning principles and a comprehensive intervention model. In *Behavior modification: Principles, issues and applications*, ed. W. E. Craighead, A. E. Kazdin, and M. J. Mahoney. Boston: Houghton Mifflin, in press.

Jeffrey, D. B., and Christensen E. R. 1972. The relative efficacy of behavior therapy, will power and no-treatment control procedures for weight loss. Paper presented at the annual meeting of the Association for Advancement of Behavior Therapy, New York, October 1972.

Jeffrey, D. B.; Christensen, E. R.; and Pappas, J. P. 1972. A case study report of a behavioral modification weight reduction group: Treatment of follow-up (*Res. & Dev. Rep. 33*). University of Utah Counseling Center, Salt Lake City, Utah.

Kanfer, F. H., and Saslow, G. 1965. Outline of interview information needed for a functional analysis; Addendum to: Behavioral analysis: An alternative to diagnostic classification. *Archs. Gen. Psychiat.* 12:529–38.

Kaplan, H. I., and Kaplan, H. S. 1957. The psychosomatic concept of obesity. *J. Nerv. Ment. Dis.* 125:181–201.

Kau, M. L., and Fischer, J. 1974. Self-modification of exercise behavior. *J. Behav. Therapy & Exp. Psychiat.* 5:213–14.

Kennedy, W. A., and Foreyt, J. P. 1968. Control of eating behavior in an obese patient by avoidance conditioning. *Psychol. Rep.* 22:571–76.

Kimble, G. A. 1961. Hilgard & Marquis' *Conditioning and Learning.* New York: Appleton-Century-Crofts.

Klein, D.; Steele, R. L.; Simon, W. E.; and Primavera, L. H. 1972. Reinforcement and weight loss in schizophrenics. *Psychol. Rep.* 30:581–82.

Krop, H.; Calhoon, B.; and Verrier, R. 1971. Modification of the "Self-concept" of emotionally disturbed children by covert reinforcement. *Behav. Therapy* 2:201–4.

Lazarus, A. A. 1971. *Behavior therapy and beyond.* New York: McGraw-Hill.

Lee, A. R. 1955. Clinical symposium: Psychological and physiological aspects of marked obesity in a young adult female. *J. Hillside Hospital* 29:203–31.

Leon, G. R., and Chamberlain, K. 1973. Emotional arousal, eating patterns, and body image as differential factors associated with varying success in maintaining a weight loss. *J. Consult. Clin. Psychol.* 40:474–80.

Levitz, L. S., and Stunkard, A. J. 1974. A therapeutic coalition for obesity: Behavior modification and patient self-help. *Am. J. Psychiat.* 131:423–27.

Lick, J., and Bootzin, R. 1971. Covert sensitization for the treatment of obesity. Paper presented at the annual meeting of the Midwestern Psychological Association, Detroit, Michigan, 1971.

Lindstrom, L. L.; Balch, P.; and Reese, S. 1975. Delivery of behavioral self-control treatments for obesity: A comparison of professional, trained and untrained paraprofessional, and telephone led therapies. Unpublished manuscript, University of Arizona.

Lutzker, S. Z., and Lutzker, J. R. 1974. A two-dimensional marital contract: Weight loss and household responsibility performance. Paper presented at the annual meeting of the Western Psychological Association, San Francisco, California, April 1974.

Mahoney, M. J. 1973. Clinical issues in self-control training. Paper presented at the annual meeting of the American Psychological Association, Montreal, August 1973.

———. 1974a. Self-reward and self-monitoring techniques for weight control. *Behav. Therapy* 5:48–57.

———. 1974b. Cognition and behavior modification. Cambridge, Mass.: Ballinger.

———. 1975a. Fat fiction. *Behav. Therapy* 6:416–18.

———. 1975b. The obese eating style: Bites, beliefs and behavior modification. *Addict. Behav.* 1:47–53.

Mahoney, M. J., and Jeffrey, D. B. 1973. Weight control procedures for the individual. Counseling and Psychological Services Research and Development Report No. 41, University of Utah.

Mahoney, M. J., and Mahoney, K. 1976*a*. Cognitive factors in weight reduction. In *Counseling methods,* ed. J. D. Krumboltz and C. E. Thoresen. New York: Holt, Rinehart & Winston.

————. 1976*b*. *Permanent weight control.* New York: Norton.

————. 1976*c*. Treatment of obesity: A clinical exploration. In *Obesity: Behavioral approaches to dietary management,* ed. B. J. Williams, S. Martin, and J. P. Foreyt. New York: Brunner/Mazel.

Mahoney, M. J.; Moura, N. G. M.; and Wade, T. C. 1973. Relative efficacy of self-reward, self-punishment, self-monitoring techniques for weight loss. *J. Consult. Clin. Psychol.* 40:404–7.

Mahoney, M. J., and Thoresen, C. E. 1974. *Self-control: Power to the person.* Monterey, California: Brooks/Cole.

Maletzky, B. M. 1973. Assisted covert sensitization: A preliminary report. *Behav. Therapy* 4:117–19.

Mann, R. A. 1972. The behavior-therapeutic use of contingency contracting to control an adult behavior problem: Weight control. *J. Appl. Behav. Anal.* 5:99–109.

————. 1973. The use of contingency contracting to facilitate durability of behavior change: Weight loss maintenance. Paper presented at the annual meeting of the American Psychological Association, Montreal, August 1973.

Manno, B. 1972. Weight reduction as a function of the timing of reinforcement in a covert aversive conditioning paradigm. *Diss. Abstr. Int.* 32(7-B):4221(abstract).

Manno, B., and Marston, A. R. 1972. Weight reduction as a function of negative covert reinforcement (sensitization) versus positive covert reinforcement. *Behav. Res. & Therapy* 10:201–07.

Mayer, J. 1968. *Obesity: Causes, cost, and control.* Englewood Cliffs, N. J.: Prentice-Hall.

McKenna, R. J. 1970. Some effects of anxiety level and food cues on the eating behavior of obese and normal subjects: A comparison of the Schachterian and psychosomatic conceptions. Unpublished doctoral dissertation, University of Connecticut, 1970.

McReynolds, W. T. 1975. Family behavior therapy for obesity: Treatment and preventative implications. Paper presented at the annual meeting of the Association for Advancement of Behavior Therapy, San Francisco, December 1975.

McReynolds, W. T.; Lutz, R. N.; Paulsen, B. K.; and Kohrs, M. B. 1976. Weight loss resulting from two behavior modification procedures with nutritionists as therapists. *Behav. Therapy* 7:283–91.

Metropolitan Life Insurance Company. 1959. New weight standards for men and women. *Stat. Bull.* 40:1–4.

Meyer, V., and Crisp, A. H. 1964. Aversion therapy in two cases of obesity. *Behav. Res. & Therapy* 2:143–47.

Meynen, G. E. 1970. A comparative study of three treatment approaches with the obese: Relaxation, covert sensitization and modified systematic desensitization. *Diss. Abstr. Int.* 31(5-B): 2998(abstract).

Mikulas, W. L. 1972. *Behavior modification: An overview.* New York: Harper & Row.

Moore, C. H., and Crum, B. C. 1969. Weight reduction in a chronic schizophrenic by means of operant conditioning procedures: A case study. *Behav. Res. & Therapy* 7:129–31.

Morganstern, K. P. 1974. Cigarette smoke as a noxious stimulus in self-managed aversion therapy for compulsive eating. *Behav. Therapy* 5:255–60.

Moss, F. A. 1924. Note on building likes and dislikes in children. *J. Exp. Psychol.* 7:475–78.

Murray, D. C., and Harrington, L. G. 1972. Covert aversive sensitization in the treatment of obesity. *Psychol. Rep.* 30:560.

Musante, G. J. 1976. The Dietary Rehabilitation Clinic: Evaluative report of a behavioral and dietary treatment of obesity. *Behav. Therapy* 7:198–204.

Newburgh, L. H. 1942. Obesity. *Archs. Intern. Med.* 70:1033–96.

Nisbett, R. E. 1972. Hunger, obesity, and ventromedial hypothalamus. *Psychol. Rev.* 79:433–53.

Pavlov, I. P. 1955. *Selected works.* Trans. S. Belsky, ed. J. Gibbons. Moscow: Foreign Languages Publishing House.

Penick, S. B.; Filion, R.; Fox, S.; and Stunkard, A. J. 1971. Behavior modification in the treatment of obesity. *Psychosom. Med.* 33:49–55.

Pliner, P.; Meyer, P.; and Blankstein, K. Responsiveness to affective stimuli by obese and normal individuals. *J. Abnorm. Psychol.* 83:74–80.

Powdermaker, H. 1973. An anthropological approach to the problem of obesity. In *The Psychology of Obesity: Dynamics and Treatment,* ed. N. Kiell. Springfield, Ill.: Charles C Thomas.

Rodin, J. 1973. Effects of distraction on performance of obese and normal subjects. *J. Comp & Physiol. Psychol.* 83:68–75.

Romanczyk, R. G. 1974. Self-monitoring in the treatment of obesity: Parameters of reactivity. *Behav. Therapy* 5:531–40.

Romanczyk, R. G.; Tracey, D. A.; Wilson, G. T.; and Thorpe, G. L. 1973. Behavioral techniques in the treatment of obesity: A comparative analysis. *Behav. Res. & Therapy* 11:629–40.

Ross, L. D. 1969. Cue- and cognition-controlled eating among obese and normal subjects. Unpublished doctoral dissertation, Columbia University, 1969.

Sachs, L. B.; Bean, H.; and Morrow, J. E. 1970. Comparison of smoking treatments. *Behav. Therapy* 1:465–72.

Sachs, L. B., and Ingram, G. L. 1972. Covert sensitization as a treatment for weight control. *Psychol. Rep.* 30:971–74.

Schachter, S. 1967. Cognitive effects on bodily functioning: Studies of obesity and eating. In *Neurophysiology and Emotions,* ed. D. Glass. New York: Rockefeller University and the Russell Sage Foundation.

———. 1971 Some extraordinary facts about obese humans and rats. *Am. Psychol.* 26:129–44.

Schachter, S.; Goldman, R.; and Gordon, A. 1968. Effects of fear, food deprivation, and obesity on eating. *J. Pers. Soc. Psychol.* 10:91–7.

Schachter, S., and Gross, L. 1968. Eating and manipulation of time. *J. Pers. Soc. Psychol.* 10:98–106.

Schopbach, R. R., and Matthews, R. A. 1945. The psychological problems in obesity. *Archs. Neurol. & Psychiat.* 54:157.

Skinner, B. F. 1969. *Contingencies of reinforcement.* New York: Appleton-Century-Crofts.

Stollak, G. E. 1967. Weight loss obtained under different experimental procedures. *Psychotherapy: Theory, Research and Practice* 4:51–64.

Stuart, R. B. 1967. Behavioral control of overeating. *Behav. Res. & Therapy* 5:337–65.

———. 1971. A three-dimensional program for the treatment of obesity. *Behav. Res. & Therapy* 9:177–86.

———. 1973. Behavioral control of overeating: A status report. Paper presented at the Fogarty International Center Conference on Obesity, Bethesda, Maryland, October 1973.

Stuart, R. B., and Davis, B. 1972a. *Slim chance in a fat world: Behavioral control of obesity.* Champaign, Ill.: Research Press.

———. 1972b. *Slim chance in a fat world: Behavioral control of obesity.* Condensed edition. Champaign, Ill.: Research Press.

Stunkard, A. J. 1958. The management of obesity. *NY State J. Med.* 58:79–87.

————. 1972. New therapies for the eating disorders. *Archs. Gen. Psychiat.* 26:391–98.

————. 1975. From exploration to action in psychosomatic medicine: The case of obesity. *Psychosom. Med.* 37:195–236.

Stunkard, A. J., and Koch, C. 1964. The interpretation of gastric motility. *Archs. Gen. Psychiat.* 2:74–82.

Stunkard, A. J., and McLaren-Hume, M. 1959. The results of treatment of obesity. *Archs. Intern. Med.* 103:79–85.

Stunkard, A. J., and Rush, J. 1974. Dieting and depression reexamined: A critical review of reports of untoward responses during weight reduction for obesity. *Ann. Intern. Med.* 81:526–33.

Swanson, D. W., and Dinello, F. 1969. Therapeutic starvation in obesity. *Diseases of the Nervous System* 30:669–74.

Thorpe, J. G.; Schmidt, E.; Brown, P. T.; and Castell, D. 1964. Aversion-relief therapy: A new method for general application. *Behav. Res. & Therapy* 2:71–82.

Tighe, T. J., and Elliott, R. 1968. A technique for controlling behavior in natural life settings. *J. Appl. Behav. Anal.* 1:263–66.

Tyler, V. O., and Straughan, J. H. 1970. Coverant control and breath holding as techniques for the treatment of obesity. *Psychol. Rec.* 20:473–78.

Upper, D., and Newton, J. G. 1971. A weight-reduction program for schizophrenic patients on a token economy unit: Two case studies. *J. Behav. Therapy & Exp. Psychiat.* 2:113–15.

U.S. Public Health Service. *Obesity and health.* Washington, D.C.: U.S. Government Printing Office, undated.

U.S. Public Health Service. 1965. *Weight, height, and selected body dimensions of adults.* Washington, D.C.: U.S. Government Printing Office.

Viernstein, L. 1968. Evaluation of therapeutic techniques of covert sensitization. Unpublished data. Charlottesville, N.C.: Queens College.

Wagner, M. K., and Bragg, R. A. Comparing behavior modification methods for habit decrement-smoking. *J. Consult. Clin. Psychol.*, in press.

Watson, D., and Tharp, R. 1972. *Self-directed behavior: Self-modification for personal adjustment.* Belmont, Calif.: Brooks/Cole.

Welsh, A. L. 1962. *Side effects of anti-obesity drugs.* Springfield, Ill.: Charles C Thomas.

Williams, R. L., and Long, J. G. 1975. *Toward a self-managed lifestyle.* Boston: Houghton Mifflin.

Wollersheim, J. P. 1970. Effectiveness of group therapy based upon learning principles in the treatment of overweight women. *J. Abnorm. Psychol.* 76:462–74.

Wolpe, J. 1954. Reciprocal inhibition as the main basis of psychotherapeutic effects. *Archs. Neurol. & Psychiat.* 72:205–26.

———. 1958. *Psychotherapy by reciprocal inhibition.* Stanford: Stanford University Press.

———. 1973. *The practice of behavior therapy.* 2d ed. New York: Pergamon.

Wolpe, J., and Lang, P. J. 1964. A fear survey schedule for use in behavior therapy. *Behav. Res. & Therapy* 2:27–30.

Wooley, S. C., and Wooley, O. W. 1973. Salivation to the sight and thought of food: A new measure of appetite. *Psychosom. Med.* 35:136–42.

Wyden, P. 1965. *The overweight society.* New York: William Morrow.